Questions and Answers for Dental Nurses

Questions and Answers for Dental Nurses

4th Edition

Carole Hollins

General Dental Practitioner, Stoke-on-Trent, England
Member of the British Dental Association
Former Chairman of the National Examining Board for Dental Nurses

WILEY Blackwell

This fourth edition first published 2022

Edition History
Blackwell Publishing Ltd. (3e, 2012)

Registered Offices
John Wiley & Sons, Inc., 111 River Street, Hoboken, NJ 07030, USA
John Wiley & Sons Ltd, The Atrium, Southern Gate, Chichester, West Sussex, PO19 8SQ, UK

Editorial Office
9600 Garsington Road, Oxford, OX4 2DQ, UK

For details of our global editorial offices, customer services, and more information about Wiley products visit us at www.wiley.com.

Wiley also publishes its books in a variety of electronic formats and by print-on-demand. Some content that appears in standard print versions of this book may not be available in other formats.

Library of Congress Cataloging-in-Publication Data Applied for

[ISBN PB: 9781119785200]

Cover Design: Wiley
Cover Image: Courtesy of Carole Hollins

Set in 10/12.5pt Sabon by Straive, Pondicherry, India
Printed and bound by CPI Group (UK) Ltd, Croydon, CR0 4YY

C9781119785200_110223

This book is dedicated to the next generation, especially Maisie, Renée and Poppy – may they all have long, happy and successful lives ahead of them.

Contents

Introduction

This fourth edition of *Questions and Answers for Dental Nurses* has been completely rewritten to accommodate the huge changes and updates that have occurred in the fields of dentistry, dental nursing and oral health since the publication of the third edition 10 years ago. The questions provided are based on the content of the textbook *Levison's Textbook for Dental Nurses 12th Edition*, which incorporates those changes and updates, in areas such as infection control and decontamination, oral health promotion and restorative dentistry, as well as legislative and regulative changes. The *Levison* textbook covers the full curriculum of the National Examining Board for Dental Nurses' (NEBDN) qualification, the National Diploma. The styles of the questions in this book follow those of the written components of the National Diploma – namely, one of five single best answer multiple choice questions (MCQs) and extended matching questions (EMQs). Full details of both question types with worked examples are given in the next section.

Students wishing to sit the National Diploma examination must first complete a course of study with a training provider accredited by NEBDN, part of which involves the full completion of the Record of Experience portfolio while in their training workplace. They may then sit the written component of the examination and, if successful at this stage, they will be eligible to undertake the practical component of the examination, the objective structured clinical examinations (OSCEs), an overview of which is also given in the next section. A pass awarded in the OSCEs will complete the National Diploma examination, and successful candidates may then proceed to apply and become registered professional dental nurses with the General Dental Council (GDC).

This book is designed to be used throughout the student's training course mainly as a revision aid for topics from each area of the curriculum, but ideally it should also become a useful resource in stimulating students' thought processes to enable them to understand those topics more fully. With the MCQs, by providing an explanation of the reason why just one answer out of the five choices is the single best option to a question, it is hoped that the student is able to consider the relevant topic from a different perspective than that of the bare facts laid out in the textbook. The format should encourage the student to apply a good depth of knowledge of the topic to the question, logically consider the five options and correctly reason which option is the best answer to that particularly worded question. The EMQs require the student to analyse the question scenario, then apply their reasoning skills to determine and match one, or more, correct answer options for that question scenario. This modern educational style of questioning is a welcome successor to the old-style MCQs that often required students to learn facts about a topic by rote.

Ideally then, students using this book while undertaking their training should become inquisitive about their areas of study and want to learn not just HOW to carry out a task but understand WHY they are carrying it out. Once qualified, this inquisitiveness will stand them in good stead to undergo regular continuing professional development within their scope of practice and become lifelong learners.

How to Use this Book

The book is divided into the four development outcomes of learning as stipulated by the GDC, with the development outcomes subdivided into a total of 13 chapters with questions covering the full NEBDN curriculum. This introduces the concept of the development outcomes to dental nurse students at an early stage and should assist them to relate their knowledge areas and activities to them. The GDC expects all registrants to undertake continuing professional development (CPD) activities throughout their career in line with these development outcomes, so upon qualification and registration it is hoped dental nurses will be well versed in the topics that each outcome covers and will be enabled to organise their own CPD accordingly.

The development outcomes are shown below.

- Development outcome A – Communication
- Development outcome B – Management and Leadership
- Development outcome C – Clinical
- Development outcome D – Professionalism.

Details of the two question styles for the National Diploma written paper as well as an overview of the practical component of the examination, the OSCEs, is given below. Students are advised to read this section in full before attempting to use the book as a revision aid so that they become fully familiar with the question styles and how to answer each one.

Multiple choice questions

The correct title for this style of question is one of five single best answer MCQ, and the important point to note is that, of the five answer options given, more than one MAY be a correct answer to a question but only one option will be the BEST answer for that particularly worded question. It is imperative that the student reads the question carefully before attempting to answer. All this style of question follows the form shown below.

- The question itself is usually a few sentences long – this is the question stem.
- The first sentence introduces the topic of the question (such as oral health, medical emergencies, consent and so on).

- The final sentence asks the specific question.
- This style of question is designed to test the application of the relevant knowledge.
- Key words or phrases are not highlighted.
- There are always five answer options.
- Only one of those five will be the 'best' option for that specific question and is therefore the correct answer in that instant.
- The answers are always homologous, that is, of the same form (so, all oral hygiene products, all restorative materials, all bacteria and so on).
- The answers are always set out alphabetically or numerically in ascending order (so from A to Z, or lowest to highest number).

It is important to note that the same five answer options could be used with several slightly different question stems, and with each one having a different single 'best' option answer – hence the importance of reading the specific question carefully.

As the question style always follows the same pattern, it is not possible for examination candidates to 'work out by elimination' or 'guess' the correct answer – they must have the relevant knowledge and understanding of the topic to be able to apply it to the specific question. Only then can the single best answer be identified.

Similarly, as an ascending alphabetical or numerical order is always followed in the answer options, the correct answer cannot be determined by counting how many times, say, option C has been an answer and therefore not choosing it again. The single best answer for each question will be at whichever option letter it falls at alphabetically or numerically only. So, it is quite feasible for an examination paper to have option C as the correct answer for every question asked, if the correct answer for each question happens to fall at option C alphabetically or numerically. Consequently, candidates are unable to guess the answer.

During the examination, candidates mark their single answer choice on an optical marking sheet for each question, by pencilling a horizontal line through a small box adjacent to their chosen answer option – A, B, C, D, or E. Only one box must be filled in for each question, otherwise the optical reader in the computer will reject that question, so candidates must take care to fully erase an answer when changing their option choice during the examination. Similarly, the box must only be filled in by pencilling a horizontal line in it – drawing a circle around the box or putting a cross through it will also cause the optical reader to reject that question.

Below are five examples of the one of five single best answer style MCQs, with the correct answer and accompanying explanation for each one.

1. The General Dental Council Standards document states that patients expect the dental team to act promptly to protect their safety if there are concerns about the health of a team member in relation to drug abuse. Which one of the following options is the term used to describe this action?

A Complaining
B Raising concerns
C Reporting untoward incidents
D Safeguarding children
E Safeguarding vulnerable adults

The correct answer is B. Any person acting under the influence of drugs can be assumed to be not of sound mind at the time, as the drugs are, by definition, mind-altering substances. The potential of the drug abuser to cause harm or injury to anyone while under the influence of drugs is huge, especially in the health environment when patients have put their trust in the professionalism of the staff treating them.

2. Dental caries, gingivitis and periodontitis are the three main dental diseases of concern to the dental team. Advice on preventing them and providing treatment when one or more diseases are present forms the bulk of the daily work of the team. Which one of the following options describes the role of fluoride in the reduction of a patient's caries experience?
   A Control bacterial plaque build-up
   B Control the host response to disease
   C Modify any contributory factors
   D Modify the diet
   E Strengthen teeth against acids

The correct answer is E. The inorganic crystal structure of teeth is composed of hydroxyapatite crystals. When fluoride is applied to teeth topically (as gels and varnishes) or is incorporated into the tooth structure from systemic fluoride (such as fluoridated water), it forms fluorapatite crystals, which is a crystalline structure more resistant to damage by weak organic acids formed in the mouth by bacteria. The stronger structure results in fewer dental cavities.

3. All student dental nurses begin their careers working in a supervised environment, either in general practice or in specialist clinics or hospitals. A specific risk assessment will have been carried out to ensure their safety within that environment while carrying out potentially hazardous work activities. Which one of the following options is the most likely activity that could result in the student dental nurse receiving a projectile injury to the eye?
   A Chairside assisting
   B Instrument decontamination
   C Use of autoclave
   D Use of chemicals
   E Use of X-rays

The correct answer is A. During use, dental handpieces revolve at a very fast speed, and it is not unusual for pieces of filling or tooth to shoot out of a patient's mouth while being drilled. All chairside staff should wear personal protective equipment specifically to protect their eyes during treatment sessions.

4. Many diseases are caused by contamination of the body cells by microscopic living organisms, collectively called pathogenic micro-organisms, or pathogens. Which one of the following pathogens are types of microscopic plant-like organisms that grow across the surface of body cells and tissues?
   A Bacteria
   B Fungi
   C Prions
   D Protozoa
   E Viruses

The correct answer is B. Microscopically, fungi are similar in appearance to colonies of mushrooms or toadstools, with an extensive network of surface branches lying across the body tissue and their reproductive bodies sprouting out like mushrooms. They are the largest of the pathogenic micro-organisms.

5. Composite filling materials are tooth-coloured restoratives that are available in a wide range of shades, enabling them to be matched to a patient's tooth colour when used. The majority are light-cured and contain an inorganic filler, resin and a catalyst that is activated when exposed to the curing light at the chairside. Which one of the following options is an example of a composite material used to avoid the need for incremental curing during restoration?
   A Bulk-fill composite
   B Hybrid composite
   C Microfine composite
   D Nano composite
   E Universal composite

The correct answer is A. Bulk-fill composites can be placed into a cavity as one increment and cured to a depth of 4–5 mm (depending on the material used) in one set. This significantly reduces the clinical time required to restore a large cavity with composite filling material, as ordinary composite materials only set to a depth of 2 mm and therefore require incremental curing, making the restorative procedure much longer to achieve.

Extended matching questions

This style of question consists of a given topic heading (such as microbiology, disease prevention, pain and anxiety control and so on) accompanied by a lead-in statement and a list of options. Each option list is followed by a set of questions that each describe a particular scenario, for which the candidate must choose one or more matching options from the list as the answer(s) to the specific question. All candidates have the same definitive option lists provided in the written examination paper for each question set and can only match answers for each question from the relevant option list. All this style of question follows the form shown below.

- The topic covered by the question set is stated, to help focus the candidate's thought processes.

- The lead-in statement explains what candidates are required to do and how many options they are required to choose from the list – this will either be 'the single most appropriate. . .' or 'the requested number of. . .'.
- The option list will usually contain a minimum of eight options.
- The options are always homologous – of the same form (so all surgical instruments, all restorative materials and so on).
- The options are always set out alphabetically or numerically in ascending order (so from a) to b) or from lowest to highest number).
- The questions are set out as several sentences that describe a detailed scenario.
- They are designed to test the candidate's analytical and reasoning skills, as well as requiring a more detailed and concise application of their knowledge.
- Key words or phrases are not highlighted.
- Each topical option list is accompanied by a question set, rather than a single question.

The candidates must read the lead-in statement carefully for each question set, as this gives the information required to match an answer to each question correctly. So, are they matching an appropriate emergency drug to a medical emergency scenario, or an appropriate oral hygiene item to an oral health assessment scenario, or an appropriate instrument to set out for a restorative procedure and so on. Also, the lead-in statement will state whether just one or more than one answer may be required for questions within that set – obviously if the wrong number is given by the candidate, the answer will be rejected. Where multiple matched answers are to be given, each question will state the number required.

Again, the alphabetical or numerical order of the option list will prevent the candidates from attempting to guess a likely answer by believing, for example, that option e) has not been used previously and so choose it. The lead-in statement for EMQs will always state that 'each option might be used once, more than once or not at all'. Candidates are required to mark their answers as a pencilled horizontal line on an optical marking sheet, as detailed above in the section on MCQs.

With EMQs, candidates are required to first understand the question scenario as it is described, then apply detailed knowledge of the topic to the scenario so that they can reason out and match the answer(s) from the option list.

Below are several examples of extended matching questions and answers showing the various formats discussed.

Topic: Head and neck anatomy

For each of the following head and neck anatomy questions, select the single most appropriate answer from the option list. Each option might be used once, more than once or not at all.

a) External carotid artery
b) Glossopharyngeal nerve
c) Internal carotid artery
d) Long buccal nerve
e) Medial pterygoid

f) Occipital bone
g) Temporal bone
h) Temporalis
i) Trigeminal nerve

1. The muscles of mastication are those running between the skull and the mandible that are responsible for closing the mouth and chewing movements. Which one of the options listed is the muscle of mastication that has a point of insertion on the coronoid process of the mandible and acts to pull this jaw backwards and closed?

The correct answer is h). Temporalis runs from the temporal bone on the side of the head, under the zygomatic arch and inserts onto the coronoid process. It can be seen bulging in the temple region when the teeth are clenched together.

2. The nerve supply to the head is extensive and supplied by the 12 pairs of cranial nerves, which leave the brain directly through the base of the skull to innervate the area. Which one of the options listed is the name of the fifth cranial nerve that supplies the majority of structures in the oral cavity?

The correct answer is i). The trigeminal nerve is the cranial nerve of most importance to the dental team, and it splits into three divisions: the ophthalmic, the maxillary and the mandibular. The mandibular division is a combination nerve as it carries both sensory and motor components.

3. The major arteries carrying oxygenated blood to the head and neck region are the common carotid arteries, which are direct branches from the arch of the aorta as it leaves the left ventricle. Which one of the options listed is the branch of the common carotid artery that supplies this oxygenated blood to the face and oral cavity?

The correct answer is a). The common carotid artery divides into two branches in the upper neck area; the external carotid artery, which runs outside the cranium and supplies the face and oral cavity, and the internal carotid artery, which passes into the brain and supplies it and some of the sensory organs, such as the eyes.

Topic: Medical emergencies – drugs and equipment

For each of the following medical emergency questions, select the single most appropriate answer from the option list. Each option might be used once, more than once or not at all.

a) Adrenaline
b) AED
c) Aspirin
d) Blood glucose monitor
e) Glucagon
f) Glucogel
g) Glyceryl trinitrate

h) Midazolam buccal
i) Needle and syringe
j) OP airway
k) Oxygen
l) Pocket face mask
m) Portable suction device
n) Pulse oximeter
o) Salbutamol
p) Sphygmomanometer

1. A collapsed patient is found in the waiting room of the dental practice by a staff member, and the alarm is raised. On checking the patient's airway, the dentist discovers the casualty's mouth contains vomit. Which one of the options listed is the item most likely to be required to immediately aid the casualty?

The correct answer is m). As the patient is located in the waiting area the mains operated surgery suction unit cannot be utilised to clear the vomit. A portable suction device is emergency equipment that should be held by all dental workplaces and is best kept with the emergency drugs kit in a centralised area of the workplace, with appropriate signage displayed for easy location.

2. Following a scale and polish procedure, a patient begins to feel unwell and complains of pains in his chest and arm. On checking his medical history record on the computer, he is found to suffer from angina and is given oxygen using a pocket face mask system. Which one of the options listed is the other item most likely to be required to assist the casualty?

The correct answer is g). Glyceryl trinitrate (GTN) spray should be held in the emergency drugs kit and should be administered to any patient suspected of having an angina attack. Patients usually carry their own supply, but that of the workplace will be in date, a full container and easily located so is best used in an emergency situation. It is sprayed under the casualty's tongue where the thin mucous membrane allows the active drug to be rapidly absorbed into the blood stream and carried to the heart. The spray can be administered several times to ease the angina symptoms, but repeat applications may indicate the casualty is veering towards a cardiac arrest.

3. A known epileptic patient has attended the practice for dental treatment but becomes unwell while having radiographs taken. The staff believe the audible alarm of the machine has triggered a seizure, and the patient continues fitting for more than 5 minutes. Which one of the options listed is the item most likely to be required to assist the casualty?

The correct answer is h). A prolonged seizure (5 minutes plus) or repeat seizures occurring without the casualty regaining consciousness indicate status epilepticus – a very serious medical emergency that requires professional support for the dental team. While awaiting paramedics, midazolam buccal gel should be administered into the buccal sulcus of the casualty by the rescuer, where it will be rapidly absorbed into the blood stream. Use the buccal sulcus closest to the floor (with the casualty lying on their side) so that the gel does not trickle into their oropharynx and cause choking.

Topic: Disease prevention and health advice

For each of the following disease prevention and health advice questions, select the requested number of most appropriate answers from the option list. Each option might be used once, more than once or not at all.

a) 1450 ppm
b) 5000 ppm
c) 22,600 ppm
d) Crowded teeth
e) Hydrogen peroxide
f) Mouth breathing
g) Sodium fluoride
h) Stannous fluoride
i) Unbalanced occlusion

1. A young mother is concerned to learn that her 5-year-old son has several areas of demineralisation and two cavities in his deciduous teeth when checked by the dentist, as she ensures his teeth are brushed twice daily with 'milk teeth' type toothpaste. The dentist explains that this type of toothpaste has too little fluoride for children over 3 years of age. Which two of the options listed are the most likely fluoride concentrations that the dentist will recommend for regular toothbrushing and use for topical fluoride applications to the child, in ppm?

The correct answers are a) and c). All children over 3 years of age should be using toothpastes with the adult concentration of fluoride at 1450 ppm, to provide the maximum level of protection to their deciduous teeth and then their permanent teeth as they erupt. At each recall appointment, the child should also have a fluoride gel applied to all his teeth to help strengthen them against further carious attack. The gels are typically a fluoride strength of 22,600 ppm.

2. Modern toothpastes contain many different constituents, and some patients may find it difficult to determine which product is best for their specific oral health needs. The dental team are well placed to advise patients about the most suitable products available for their particular needs, depending whether they require products to combat dental caries or periodontal disease. Which two of the options listed are constituents that may be found in a toothpaste designed to protect against caries and relieve sensitivity?

The correct answers are g) and h). Fluoride is the ingredient present to protect against dental caries, and many toothpastes contain it as sodium fluoride at

1450 ppm. Stannous fluoride is present in some 'sensitivity' toothpastes to help reduce the electric shock-type sensation that some patients experience with cold drinks, foods or when breathing in cold air.

Objective Structured Clinical Examination

For the sake of completeness, an overview of the practical element of the National Diploma examination is given here to assist candidates in readying themselves for the final part of the examination. More detailed information is given in the textbook *Levison's Textbook for Dental Nurses 12th Edition.* The OSCEs are usually held several weeks after each round of written examinations has been completed, with only those candidates who pass the written section being eligible to then enter for the OSCEs.

The OSCEs provide an accurate and fair assessment of all candidates while carrying out various practical or clinical tasks. As the full name suggests, the examination style is both objective and structured in the way that candidates are assessed while undertaking OSCEs. The examiner does not ask any questions of the candidate during each section of the examination (so they are objective and not subjective, or rather, not based on the examiner's opinion after having asked the candidate any random questions), and the examiner grades each candidate's practical/clinical performance against set criteria as they carry out the required task. The set criteria are exactly the same for every candidate at whichever examination centre they attend and are followed by every examiner, so the OSCEs are a structured examination.

Each examination sitting will have up to 15 OSCE stations that every candidate must go through, and they are usually timed at 5 minutes each. Other than to welcome candidates to each test area and ask if they have read the 'candidate instructions' for the individual test beforehand, the examiner does not speak to the candidate but merely observes their performance within the 5-minute timing.

There are four general types of practical assessment that the OSCEs will cover, and each is designed to test both the professional and practical skills of the candidate.

- Communication skills – such as giving specific oral hygiene advice or post-operative advice to a patient (the patient will be a professional actor)
- Medical emergency – such as an asthma attack scenario with a professional actor as the patient
- Mixing skills – any dental material from within the NEBDN curriculum
- Clinical skills – such as setting up instruments for a certain procedure or completing a charting exercise.

The candidate instructions will state the scenario relevant to the OSCE station, and the candidate is able to read these instructions before the 5-minute timing starts. The instructions will be clear and concise, so that the task to be carried out by the candidate will be obvious to them. Where a patient (actor) is involved in the scenario, the candidate will be scored objectively by both the examiner and the patient for that OSCE station.

To ensure that every candidate is assessed objectively, the following system is strictly followed.

- Every examination centre will carry out exactly the same OSCE assessments, using exactly the same resources.
- All candidates and patient instructions will be worded exactly the same, in every examination centre.
- All candidates will be marked against the same performance criteria and in the same way, as the examiners have been trained and calibrated to each other.
- All candidates will rotate through the OSCE stations in a set order until they have completed the full cycle.
- A single timer is used for each cycle of stations (usually a bell), so candidates cannot have too little, or too much, time at any station.
- All candidates are allowed 1 minute to read the scenario and candidate instructions for each station, before entering the station and beginning the assessment when the bell rings.
- No candidate is allowed to enter the station until the start of the 5-minute assessment period.
- The candidate may repeat the assessment within the 5-minute time period if they wish.
- The examiner will not ask any questions of the candidate.
- Candidates may carry out a practical task while talking their way through it if they wish (some candidates may find this helps to focus their actions), but they will only be assessed on the performance criteria listed on the examiner mark sheet and not on anything they say.
- There are no 'killer' stations, where the candidate must pass that one station or be failed for the whole OSCE examination.

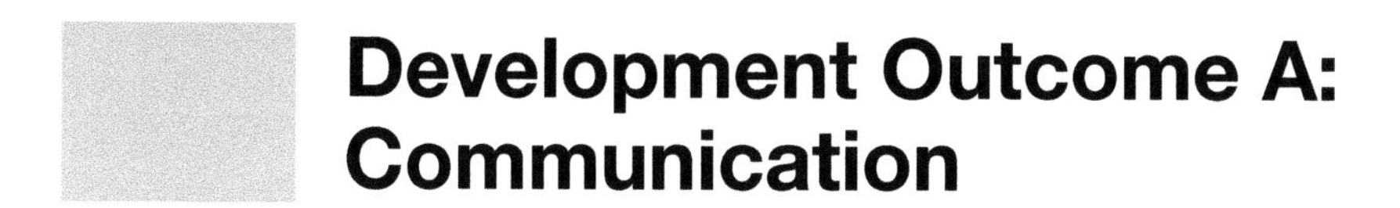

Development Outcome A: Communication

1 Communication Skills

Multiple choice questions

1. Most dental workplaces will treat patients of a wide age range, from young children to elderly pensioners, and the communication skills required by the team to treat each group successfully varies greatly. Which one of the following options is the least likely communication skill to achieve successful toothbrushing compliance by a primary school-age child?
   A Able to ask questions of team
   B Appropriate vocabulary for age
   C Describing likely dental treatment
   D Hands-on teaching technique
   E Use of physical aids to teach

2. The act of communicating with someone is to give or exchange information with them, and this can be done both verbally and non-verbally. Which one of the following non-verbal communication actions would indicate that the listener is indeed listening to the speaker?
   A Breaking eye contact
   B Continuing another task
   C Facing them
   D Interrupting them
   E Turning from them

3. During a dental appointment, patients are often provided with a lot of information by the dental team: oral health advice, treatment advice, discussions of treatment options, etc. Sometimes it may be difficult for them to clearly remember all that has been mentioned. Which one of the following options is the preferred method of reinforcing the information so that the patient remembers it?
   A Ask a colleague to repeat it
   B Ask the dentist to repeat it
   C Provide it in written format

Questions and Answers for Dental Nurses, Fourth Edition. Carole Hollins.

D Repeat it at the next appointment
E Repeat it during the appointment

4. From time to time the dental team will provide treatment for patients with a disability such as reduced vision or partial sightedness. Good communication skills by the team are important in ensuring that these patients receive treatment in a safe manner and are comfortable doing so. Which one of the following options is the least likely communicative action to assist partially sighted or blind patients to undergo dental treatment?
   A Describe likely sensations
   B Describe likely sounds
   C Play music during treatment session
   D Provide information in Braille
   E Use magnifiers for written information

5. Good communication skills are of great importance in encouraging patients to take an active role in managing their own oral and general health. If the person advising them has poor communication skills, the patient is unlikely to follow the advice. Which one of the following options would indicate communicators have good communication skills when advising a patient?
   A Butting in verbally
   B Folding their arms
   C Rolling their eyes
   D Sitting down
   E Turning away

6. The requirement for the dental team to communicate effectively with patients is enshrined in the General Dental Council (GDC) Standards document. Which one of the following options is the specific core ethical principle of professionalism in this document that deals with the issue of communication skills?
   A Principle 1
   B Principle 2
   C Principle 3
   D Principle 4
   E Principle 5

7. In modern dental workplaces, patients often receive various stages of treatment and oral healthcare from several members of the dental team throughout the delivery of a treatment plan. It is therefore important that all team members give the same messages so that the patient does not become confused. Which one of the following options is the most likely method used by the team to avoid giving conflicting advice to patients?
   A Copy what the dentist says
   B 'Google' the topic
   C Have a written protocol

D Learn the message by rote
E Refer to a textbook

8. Many dental workplaces deliver oral healthcare and treatment to patients in a multiracial society and for many of those patients, English is not their first language. It is important that patients understand the information they are given, otherwise they cannot give valid consent for treatment. Which one of the following options is the least effective method of giving dental information to a non-English-speaking patient?
   A Allow family to interpret
   B Issue relevant NHS leaflet
   C Talk slowly
   D Use 'Language Line' service
   E Use suitable online translation

9. From time to time the dental team will provide treatment for patients with a disability such as hearing loss or profound deafness. Good communication skills by the team are important in ensuring that these patients receive treatment in a safe manner and are comfortable doing so. Which one of the following options is the least effective method of communicating with a partially deaf patient?
   A Remove mask while talking
   B Shout instructions
   C Sit facing patient while talking
   D Use hearing loop device
   E Write down information

10. Most dental workplaces will treat patients of a wide age range, from young children to elderly pensioners, and the communication skills required by the team to treat each group successfully vary greatly. Which one of the following options is a patient age range that is most likely to respond to receiving oral health advice in short interactive sessions?
    A Pensioners
    B Primary school
    C Teenagers
    D Toddlers
    E University students

11. Sometimes, despite the best efforts of the dental team, the ability to communicate the detrimental effects of patients' habits or actions on their oral and general health fails. Patients have the right to make their own decisions, of course, in all matters concerning their own oral and general health, and the dental team must respect this. Which one of the following options is the most likely communication method to impress an otherwise non-receptive patient?
    A Accept defeat and give no further advice
    B Provide relevant statistics
    C Relay success of other patients

D Reprimand the patient
E Show a relevant photograph

12. Good communication skills are required by all members of the dental team when dealing with patients, to ensure that the patients can give consent for any treatment proposed by the team. Which one of the following options is an example of a team member showing good communication skills when dealing with a patient?
A Giving no information
B Leaving questions unanswered
C Speaking a different language
D Using clinical pictures
E Using dental terminology

13. Good communication between the dental team and their patients is crucial in providing relevant oral and general health information, for the benefit of the patients. Which one of the following options is an example of verbal communication?
A Discussing a treatment plan
B Giving an information leaflet
C Listening to a complaint
D Making eye contact
E Smiling at the patient

Extended matching questions

For each of the following communication skills questions, select the single most appropriate answer from the option list. Each option might be used once, more than once or not at all.

a) Break eye contact
b) Face patient
c) Face-to-face session
d) Group session
e) Language line
f) Provide information in Braille
g) Roll their eyes
h) Use hearing loop
i) Use leaflets

1. A teenager attends the practice as an emergency and is diagnosed with acute necrotising ulcerative gingivitis. Following emergency treatment and then a thorough scaling, the patient will require oral hygiene instruction with regard to effective cleaning and possibly smoking cessation advice. Which one of the options listed is likely to be the most effective way of giving the advice to this patient?

2. Following the Covid-19 pandemic of 2020, your workplace has installed a permanent glass barrier at reception to ensure the safety of staff while carrying out administrative duties, by preventing patients and visitors from encroaching into their personal space while at reception. Unfortunately, several elderly patients with hearing aids now find it hard to understand what is being said to them through the glass pane, as voices are muffled. Which one of the options listed is a technique of assisting sound transmission for these patients?

3. While closing down the surgery at the end of a clinical session, a member of staff forgot to run the disinfectant solution through the aspiration unit to clean it. The following morning the equipment was found not to be working correctly as the debris of the previous day had solidified in the pipework. Which one of the options listed is a non-verbal communication action that indicates the member of staff responsible for the breakdown is unconcerned about the issue when challenged by the employer?

4. A patient has returned to the practice weeks after having a set of dentures fitted, complaining that they are still very loose and that they fall out when she tries to eat. Having had the dentures adjusted several times, she is demanding to have a full refund as she says the dentures are not fit for purpose. Which one of the options listed is the correct non-verbal communication action to take in this situation?

5. The practice has organised an open day to coincide with the National Smile Week, and a local Brownies club are to attend for an organised visit. Which one of the options listed is likely to be the most effective way of providing simple oral hygiene information in this circumstance?

Answers

Multiple choice questions

1. *The correct answer is C.* Describing possible dental treatment that may be necessary if children do not brush their teeth regularly and effectively, especially if words such as 'toothache', 'smelly breath' and 'needle' are used, is usually quite counter-productive. Indeed, it may seem threatening to some patients. Instead, the dental team should engage children in correct brushing activities, in a friendly manner and at a communication level appropriate to their age. At this age children tend to respond well to a hands-on, getting-involved approach to instruction.

2. *The correct answer is C.* Facing someone while they speak indicates the listener is actually listening to them, whereas most of the other options indicate the listener has mentally dismissed the speaker and is concentrating on something else. Interrupting someone while they speak, apart from being rude, also indicates the listener believes what they have to say is more important or that they disagree with what the speaker is saying.

3. *The correct answer is C.* Pre-written templates for advice, such as post-operative instructions, or information leaflets about a new type of treatment are invaluable in reinforcing important information from the dental team to their patients. Patients should be encouraged to take the written information away and read it at their leisure so that they then follow advice correctly or understand proposed treatments better, or it prompts them to ask further questions to clarify the information.

4. *The correct answer is C.* Although usually relaxing to most patients and staff (depending on the music played), any background noise may hinder partially sighted or blind patients from relaxing during a treatment session, as it makes it more difficult for them to hear the likely sounds they have been told to expect during the treatment. Instead, the clinician is far better providing almost a running commentary of the treatment as it progresses through the session, and this also helps to reinforce the patient's trust in the team and that they are totally focussed on the patient.

5. *The correct answer is D.* Sitting down while talking to someone, or while they are talking to you, indicates that they have your attention – they are being listened to and communicated with. All other options are examples of poor communication skills and that the person is being dismissive, defensive or not believing what is being said.

6. *The correct answer is B.* The GDC Standards document says that the whole dental team must demonstrate good communication skills so that patients can understand what is being said to them, otherwise they cannot be said to have given consent for treatment. The document also says the team should listen to their patients, take their individual needs into consideration and promote their rights and responsibilities to make decisions about their health and care.

7. *The correct answer is C.* Written protocols do not require to be learned and repeated from memory; they are always available to be referred to while talking to the patient. Their content will not change between patients or appointments and will therefore remain consistent. In addition, protocols are developed and produced by the dental team together, often during discussions at staff meetings, so the information given will have been accepted and agreed upon by all team members.

8. *The correct answer is C.* If patients do not speak English it is irrelevant whether they are spoken to quickly or slowly – they will not understand either way. Non-English NHS information leaflets, 'Language Line' and online translation software are all excellent methods of ensuring that all patients understand the information they are being given by the dental team and are therefore able to give consent. Interpretation by a family member is acceptable in some situations but is reliant on the knowledge level of the interpreter – often younger family members (even children) are relied on to impart sometimes complicated health information to an older family member. This is not an ideal situation.

9. *The correct answer is B.* Partially deaf patients quite rightly become fed up with everyone shouting at them, believing this helps to impart information to them more effectively. Instead, many subconsciously lip read when they are being spoken to, so being able to watch a speaker's mouth while they are talking is very important to them. Facing the patient and especially removing a mask while talking, using clear enunciation of words and talking at a regular speed all enable the team to communicate effectively with partially deaf patients. Hearing loops at enclosed reception desks are useful for patients wearing a hearing aid and, if all else fails, providing information in a suitable written format ensures a level of communication with the patient.

10. *The correct answer is B.* Primary school children have short attention spans but are never happier than if they can physically take part in an activity. Good examples of dental relevance are arranging stacks of food and drink packaging as 'good' and 'bad' for teeth, toothbrushing sessions (especially if disclosed by a member of the team first, and with aprons on), relevant drawing and colouring activities and so on.

11. *The correct answer is E.* As the saying goes, 'a picture paints a thousand words', and although some clinical photographs may be used as a shock tactic, sometimes it is what is necessary to convey information. With gingivitis, poor oral hygiene, periodontitis and caries, if the photograph is actually of the patient's own mouth and shown in a sensitive rather than accusatory manner, it is often the only way of convincing the patient that change is required.

12. *The correct answer is D.* Rather than trying to describe, for example, what a crown is and how the treatment is carried out, show the patient before and after photographs of a successful case. This allows patients to visualise the improvement achieved with the treatment and relate it to themselves. It allows them to ask further questions about the procedure, and their understanding can be enhanced by the provision of further written information too.

13. *The correct answer is A.* When a treatment plan has been formulated it must be discussed verbally with the patient so that the patient can accept the proposed treatment and give consent, or refuse part or all of the treatment plan and give limited or no consent, respectively. During the discussion the patient must be told of alternative treatments where appropriate, the risks and benefits of the proposed treatment, the consequences of not having the treatment where appropriate and the costs of the treatment.

Extended matching questions

1. *The correct answer is c).* Teenagers often go through a phase of being embarrassed about their bodies, especially as they go through puberty and mature. They do not respond well to being ridiculed or admonished in front of parents or siblings and may tend to show off and 'act up' in front of friends or girlfriends/boyfriends. It is best to provide their oral hygiene instruction away from others, in a face-to-face session where they can ask questions without appearing silly and where difficult topics such as smoking can be discussed without others overhearing.

2. *The correct answer is h).* Modern hearing aids have switches that enable normal sound to be received differently when activated around a hearing loop device. When in use, amplified background noise is blocked while speech is transmitted clearly so the patient and reception staff can converse normally through the glass.

3. *The correct answer is g).* Eye rolling when being confronted about an issue indicates a lack of care or interest by the person being challenged. It can be interpreted as almost saying 'so what?' or 'not again?' by the challenger and is rude, dismissive and inflammatory.

4. *The correct answer is b).* Facing someone while they are talking to you indicates that you are listening to what they say and they have your attention. It is polite to do so and can often diffuse a tense situation.

5. *The correct answer is d).* When a group of individuals, especially of a similar age, require oral hygiene instruction and information it is best to provide it in a group session. That way, everyone is engaged and occupied at the same time so that no one is left out and no one becomes bored.

1a Consent and Record Keeping

Multiple choice questions

1. One of the requirements of gaining valid consent from patients is to ensure that they understand the decisions they are being asked to make about their dental care and treatment. Which one of the following options is the most efficient technique of showing that a patient has the necessary understanding of the proposed treatment?
   A Pay for the treatment
   B Repeat back the information they have been given
   C Sign a consent form
   D Tell their family about the treatment
   E Undergo the treatment

2. The issue of consent is a complicated one but of great importance to the dental team. All team members must have a suitable understanding of the issue to allow them to work in line with the GDC's Standards requirements of the dental professions. Which one of the following options is the term used to describe consent that has been given by the patient without coercion or threat from another person?
   A Ability
   B Informed
   C Specific
   D Valid
   E Voluntary

3. To give informed consent the patient must be deemed competent to give it and have the mental capacity to show understanding of the situation. Which one of the following options is not a requirement for a patient to be deemed competent and have mental capacity?
   A Ability to verbally agree or disagree
   B Understand consequences of declining treatment
   C Understand consequences of having treatment

Questions and Answers for Dental Nurses, Fourth Edition. Carole Hollins.

D Understand treatment is required
E Understand what is wrong

4. To be able to give consent for their own treatment, patients must be deemed competent to do so and have the mental capacity to show they have a full understanding of the situation. In some circumstances a patient may be deemed to be 'Gillick competent' and therefore able to give consent. Which one of the following options is the group of patients most likely to be deemed 'Gillick competent'?
   A Child to age of 16 years
   B Competent adult
   C Holder of Lasting Power of Attorney
   D Parent of child to 16 years
   E Patient 16–18 years old

5. The ability of others to give consent for treatment on behalf of a patient is enshrined in the Mental Capacity Act 2005 Code of Practice. Which one of the following options is the main principle that all those acting on behalf of someone deemed incompetent must follow, in line with this Act?
   A Access minimal care whenever possible
   B Access NHS care whenever possible
   C Acquire most cost-effective treatment
   D Act in best interests of patient
   E Keep appointment times

6. The Data Protection Act 1998 was updated in 2018 to include the General Data Protection Regulations (GDPR). These require organisations to be more accountable in the way they collect, use, store and dispose of personal information. Which one of the following options is the main aim of the GDPR?
   A Allow data access between hospitals
   B Allow data access between primary and secondary care
   C Encourage market research
   D Prevent data being destroyed
   E Prevent data being shared without consent

7. Patient records may be kept as hard (paper) copies, as digital records on a computer or as a combination of both. Whichever method is used, they must be written at the time of seeing the patient or as soon as possible after, so that they are in date order. Which one of the following options is the correct term for this particular requirement?
   A Accurate
   B Comprehensive
   C Contemporaneous
   D Data protection
   E Probity

8. As all members of the dental team have access to, and deal with, patient information on a daily basis, it is a requirement under the General Data Protection Regulations (GDPR) 2018 that all healthcare personnel understand the regulations and how to comply with them. Which one of the following options is the section of GDPR that explains the procedure to be followed by the workplace when patients wish to read their own dental records?
   A Consent
   B Individual rights
   C Lawful basis
   D Privacy
   E Subject access request

9. Occasionally a dental workplace may have more than one patient with the same first name and surname. It is vitally important that two patients and their records do not become mixed up, otherwise incorrect or inappropriate treatment, non-referral or wrong charges may occur. Which one of the following options is the minimum amount of information that should be checked with patients to confirm their correct identity?
   A Name, address, clinician
   B Name, address, date of birth
   C Name, clinician, date of birth
   D Name, clinician, reason for attendance
   E Name, reason for attendance

10. The Data Protection Act 1998 was updated in 2018 with the introduction of the General Data Protection Regulations (GDPR). Their aim is to protect the confidentiality of sensitive personal data held at the workplace, including dental and health records. Which one of the following is the medico-legally recommended length of time that dental records of adult patients should be retained by the workplace before they are securely destroyed?
    A 2 years
    B 6 years
    C 11 years
    D 25 years
    E Never destroyed

11. Patients have the right of access to their own manual or computerised medical and dental records written since November 1991, under the Data Protection Act 1998, the General Data Protection Regulations (GDPR) 2018 and the Access to Health Records Act 1990. Strict provisos are in place to ensure the release of these records is carried out appropriately. Which one of the following options is not a requirement for the correct release of a patient's dental records?
    A Data controller must approve access
    B Data controller must respond within 1 month
    C Dental terminology must be explained on request

D Patient must pay an administration fee
E Patient request must be made in writing

12. As all members of the dental team have access to, and deal with, patient information on a daily basis it is a requirement under the General Data Protection Regulations (GDPR) 2018 that all healthcare personnel understand the regulations and how to comply with them. Which one of the following options is the section of GDPR that explains how a patient's information is shared with others?
A Consent
B Individual rights
C Lawful basis
D Privacy
E Subject access request

13. Under the General Data Protection Regulations 2018 the dental workplace must identify the legal reason for which it holds information about both staff and patients. There are six legal bases identified, and one or more of these must be stated for each area of information held. Which one of the following options is the legal basis for NHS workplaces to hold statistical information about their patients, such as how many fall into a certain age range?
A Consent
B Contractual
C Legal obligation
D Legitimate interest
E Public interest

Extended matching questions

For each of the following consent and record keeping questions, select the single most appropriate answer from the option list. Each option might be used once, more than once or not at all.

a) Access to Health Records 1990
b) Consent
c) Contractual
d) Data Protection Act 1998
e) Freedom of Information Act 2000
f) General Data Protection Regulations 2018
g) Legal obligation
h) Legitimate interest
i) Mental Capacity Act 2005
j) Public interest

1. Under the General Data Protection Regulations 2018, all dental workplaces must state the lawful basis for holding personal information about both their patients and their staff. Which one of the options listed is the lawful basis under which a dental workplace holds patients' addresses so that appointment reminders can be sent out in a timely manner?

2. When an adult patient dies, the dental workplace is obliged to hold onto their records for a minimum amount of time before securely destroying them. Medico-legally the workplace is advised to maintain the records for 10 years after the patient's last attendance (so 11 years in total). Which one of the options listed is the Act that allows a relevant person to receive copies of these records when requested?

3. The Information Commissioner's Office (ICO) produced a document titled 'GDPR: 12 Steps to Take Now' to assist all workplaces to become compliant with the new regulations. One of the steps advises how the dental workplace can use the data they hold about their patients for marketing purposes, stating that patients must 'opt in' to receive marketing information from the workplace, and that the workplace must also have permission to use a patient's image or testimonial in any marketing they undertake. Which one of the options listed is the term used in the ICO document that explains this step?

4. Under the General Data Protection Regulations 2018, all dental workplaces must state the lawful basis for holding personal information about both their patients and their staff. Which one of the options listed is the lawful basis under which the workplace can hold the National Insurance numbers of all its employees?

5. Sometimes a situation arises in the healthcare sector where it is considered in the public's interest for statistical information to be released, such as the number of pre-school children requiring dental extractions due to caries in fluoridated and non-fluoridated areas of the country. Which one of the options listed is the Act under which these types of requests can be made by a person, an organisation or the media?

Answers

Multiple choice questions

1. *The correct answer is B.* If patients can correctly repeat the information they have been given by the dental team at the end of a discussion and after having had the opportunity to ask questions, then it is safe to assume they have understood the treatment proposal. Obviously, stating information to them and having the patient repeat it back verbatim immediately is not the same and does not indicate any level of understanding of that information.

2. *The correct answer is E.* Patients alone must make the decision to proceed with any treatment proposed, without anyone trying to influence their decision one way or another. The only exceptions to the patient alone giving consent are when a parent or guardian acts on behalf of a child, or when a vulnerable adult is deemed not competent to give consent under the strict Code of Practice of the Mental Capacity Act 2005.

3. *The correct answer is A.* Patients can communicate their decision in other ways than by speech; such as people recovering from a stroke who have lost the power of speech being able to nod or shake their head or to write down their decision. They must have the ability to communicate their decision somehow, but it does not have to be verbally.

4. *The correct answer is A.* Usually consent for treatment for a child under 16 years of age would be given by a parent or guardian, but some children under this age are mature and intelligent enough to be able to give their own valid consent – this is called 'Gillick competence'. 'Gillick competence' is accepted by law as the right of a child under 16 years of age to make decisions about treatment that cannot be overruled by the parent or guardian. It applies in England and Wales, and there is a Scottish equivalent.

5. *The correct answer is D.* Whether the person giving consent is a parent, guardian, carer or Lasting Power of Attorney (or Welfare Power of Attorney in Scotland), all have a duty of care to the patient to make decisions that are always in their best interests under the Mental Capacity Act.

6. *The correct answer is E.* Previous to the introduction of GDPR it was commonplace for organisations to sell personal information to third parties for marketing, research and financial gain. For example, insurance companies holding clients' dates of birth could sell the information to an organisation marketing holidays for elderly people, who would then contact these clients out of the blue with offers of tailored holidays for their age group. Apart from the annoyance of these 'cold calls', the clients had also not given permission for their details to be passed on in this way – it was a breach of their privacy that GDPR is aimed at preventing in future.

7. *The correct answer is C.* By definition, the word contemporaneous means 'existing during or happening during the same period of time', and while it is not always possible to write notes immediately after a patient leaves the surgery, they must be written that day at the latest, otherwise their accuracy will depend on the memory of the operator alone.

8. *The correct answer is E.* The workplace should hold subject access request templates for patients to make a written request to access their records. The information must be provided by the workplace within 1 month of receiving the written request, and the patient cannot usually be charged for the cost of printing, photocopying, postage, etc. by the workplace.

9. *The correct answer is B.* While two patients with the same first and last names does happen, the likelihood of them having the same date of birth too is highly improbable. In small dental workplaces there may only be one clinician (so every patient will be seeing that clinician), and the list of reasons for attendance will be limited too.

10. *The correct answer is C.* Although NHS regulations allow dental records to be retained for just 2 years (6 years in Northern Ireland), medico-legally an adult's records should be retained for 11 years and a child's for the same or to the age of 25 years old – whichever is the longer. The Data Protection Act and the GDPR stipulate that data must be kept for no longer than is necessary.

11. *The correct answer is D.* Since the GDPR were introduced in 2018, data controllers (the 'owners' of the records) are not allowed to charge the patient an administration fee to copy the records. The only exception to this is if the request is deemed to be excessive – such as making several requests for the same information.

12. *The correct answer is B.* Under GDPR patients have various individual rights in relation to their dental records, including how the workplace shares their information with others, such as when referring them for second opinions or for hospital care. The actual process undertaken for data sharing should be laid out in the workplace's Records Management policy, their GDPR policy and their Confidentiality policy.

13. *The correct answer is E.* Under the Freedom of Information Act a request can be made to any public organisation (such as the NHS) to release statistical information that they hold, such as the numbers of certain procedures performed annually, or the length of wait on a hospital list for a procedure, etc. However, it does not allow for the release of any personal information about patients so an individual cannot be identified from the request.

Extended matching questions

1. *The correct answer is h).* The workplace must be able to contact their patient base for reasons such as this so that the business can continue to function. If patients leave no address, the workplace would have to wait until the patient contacted them before an appointment could be booked. Similarly, the workplace would be unable to advise patients of holiday closures or changes to opening times, events that could cause considerable inconvenience to all.

2. *The correct answer is a).* There is an equivalent statute for access to a deceased patient's records in Northern Ireland – the Access to Health Records (Northern Ireland) Order 1993.

3. *The correct answer is b).* This is a separate entity from a patient giving consent for treatment, where it must be informed, specific and given by the patient or the guardian/carer to be valid. Consent in relation to marketing of the dental workplace should be a signed statement by patients agreeing that they are 'opting in' to receive marketing information or are giving their written permission for the workplace to reproduce information about them in their marketing literature that would allow others to identify the patient.

4. *The correct answer is g).* The workplace must abide by tax laws and the requirements of Her Majesty's Revenue and Customs (HMRC) to operate a salary and wages system for its employees. This is a legal obligation to ensure that all personnel are paying the correct amount of tax and National Insurance to the government.

5. *The correct answer is e).* The information released is often used to highlight issues of inequality or safety but cannot contain any personal information about the persons or patients involved. Only statistical information can be released.

2 Complaints Handling

Multiple choice questions

1. Since 2015 all health and social care organisations must carry out a proper investigation and take corrective actions when care and treatment has gone wrong, and they are expected to be honest and keep the patient fully informed and supported throughout the process. Which one of the following options is the correct term for this requirement?
   A Communication procedure
   B Complaints handling procedure
   C Complaints policy
   D Duty of candour
   E Duty of care

2. The General Dental Council requires all dental workplaces to have an in-house patient complaint handling procedure in place, which should aim to fully resolve all complaints in a satisfactory and timely manner. Which one of the following options is the term used for the staff member delegated to ensure the procedure is followed correctly throughout?
   A Complaints manager
   B Investigator
   C Ombudsman
   D Responsible person
   E Supervisor

3. A complaint is any expression of dissatisfaction by a patient about the service or treatment they have received, either within the dental workplace or when in communication with staff members. Which one of the following options is an action that the workplace must take once a complaint has been received?
   A Accept liability
   B Acknowledge receipt by the month end
   C Apologise unreservedly

D Provide details of the staff member involved
E Report back to the patient by the timeline

4. Once a complaint has been successfully resolved by following the in-house patient complaint handling procedure, the full written records of the whole incident must be retained by the workplace. Which one of the following options should be carried out with these records?
   A Sent to Care Quality Commission
   B Sent to General Dental Council
   C Shredded after 1 year
   D Stored in central complaints file
   E Stored in patient's records

5. The General Dental Council requires all dental workplaces to have an in-house patient complaint handling procedure in place, which should aim to fully resolve all complaints in a satisfactory and timely manner. The procedure should be followed upon receipt of every complaint to ensure each is handled in a consistent fashion. Which one of the following options should be the final action to be taken by the dental workplace when a complaint has been made?
   A Acknowledge receipt
   B Investigate complaint
   C Provide appeals information
   D Send written report
   E Set timescale

6. Many patients do not make a complaint because they wish to receive financial compensation but to receive an apology and an explanation of the event that generated the complaint. Which one of the following options is the most important aspect of a valid complaint in terms of the dental workplace and the team?
   A Determine possible redress
   B Find out how event occurred
   C Find out what happened
   D Lay blame where relevant
   E Learn lessons to prevent recurrence

7. In the interests of good governance, the Care Quality Commission expect the dental workplace to give their patients the opportunity to comment on the care and service they have received by the dental team, whether it was a good experience or not. Which one of the following options is the least acceptable method of providing such comments?
   A Complete a satisfaction survey
   B Contact Care Quality Commission
   C Post comments on social media
   D Provide testimonials
   E Provide written feedback

8. The General Dental Council (GDC) requires all dental workplaces to have an in-house patient complaint handling procedure in place, which should aim to fully resolve all complaints in a satisfactory and timely manner. The procedure should be followed upon receipt of every complaint to ensure each is handled in a consistent fashion. Which one of the following options should be the second action to be taken by the dental workplace when a complaint has been made?
   A Acknowledge receipt
   B Investigate complaint
   C Provide appeals information
   D Send written report
   E Set timescale

9. When a patient has made a complaint to the dental workplace's in-house system and the matter has been investigated and closed, the patient may still feel unsatisfied and wish to take the matter further as a formal complaint. Which one of the following options is the organisation to whom NHS patients should complain in the first instance?
   A Care Quality Commission
   B Commissioning body
   C Dental Complaints Service
   D General Dental Council
   E Health Service Ombudsman

10. Once a complaint has been received by the dental workplace, a written acknowledgement of its receipt must be sent to the patient with an indication of the next steps to be taken and a timescale for a response. The matter must then be investigated. Which one of the following options should not form part of the investigation?
   A Admission of liability
   B Checking of written records
   C Interview with complainant
   D Interview with staff involved
   E Meeting with complainant and staff involved

11. The General Dental Council requires all dental workplaces to have an in-house patient complaint handling procedure in place, which should aim to fully resolve all complaints in a satisfactory and timely manner. The procedure should be followed upon receipt of every complaint to ensure each is handled in a consistent fashion. Which one of the following options should be the first action to be taken by the dental workplace when a complaint has been made?
   A Acknowledge receipt
   B Investigate complaint
   C Provide appeals information
   D Send written report
   E Set timescale

12. When a complaint has been fully investigated and found to be valid, it is usual procedure to reimburse the patient's costs or offer free replacement treatment as a goodwill gesture, under legislation that covers the provision of services to customers (patients). Which one of the following options is the relevant legislation in these cases?
    - A Access to Health Records Act 1990
    - B Consumer Rights Act 2015
    - C Freedom of Information Act 2000
    - D General Data Protection Regulations 2018
    - E Health and Social Care Act 2008

13. The General Dental Council requires all dental workplaces to have an in-house patient complaint handling procedure in place, which should aim to fully resolve all complaints in a satisfactory and timely manner. Which one of the following options is not a requirement of this in-house procedure?
    - A Contact details for higher authorities
    - B Display number of complaints resolved
    - C Name of complaints manager
    - D On display in reception area
    - E Written in plain language

14. The requirement for the dental team to have a clear and effective complaints procedure in place is enshrined in the General Dental Council (GDC) Standards document. Which one of the following options is the specific core ethical principle of professionalism in this document that deals with the issue of complaints and complaints handling?
    - A Principle 1
    - B Principle 3
    - C Principle 5
    - D Principle 7
    - E Principle 9

Extended matching questions

For each of the following complaints handling questions, select the single most appropriate answer from the option list. Each option might be used once, more than once or not at all.

a) Acknowledgement
b) Appeal
c) Investigation
d) Records
e) Report
f) Responsibility
g) Timescale

1. A patient has made a complaint to the dental workplace after stating he tripped on a loose piece of carpet in the waiting room and sprained his wrist while preventing himself from falling. The complaints manager has written to the patient denying the complaint and refusing a refund, as the incident was unwitnessed. Which one of the options listed is the stage of the complaints procedure that should be followed by the dissatisfied patient?

2. In line with the complaints handling policy of the dental workplace, information should be on display so that a patient is aware of the name of the person to whom they should address a complaint. Which one of the options listed is the stage of the complaints procedure that requires this information to be available?

3. During an in-house complaints procedure, conclusions will be reached that either there is no basis for the complaint, or that no blame is attributable, or that blame is attributable. Which one of the options listed is the stage of the complaints procedure that should state this information?

4. A patient has made a written complaint stating that she is unhappy with the new upper denture recently provided by the dental practice as it is very loose and tends to fall out when she is speaking. She has requested a full refund of the cost of the denture but 3 weeks later has had no response from the practice, so decides to complain to the Commissioning body instead. Which one of the options listed is the stage of the complaints procedure that the practice has failed to abide by?

5. While following the in-house complaints procedure, a patient is invited into the dental workplace to discuss an issue with the complaints manager following her complaint of a staff member being rude to her after she arrived late for a previous treatment appointment, due to heavy traffic. Which one of the options listed is the stage of the complaints procedure that is being undertaken in this scenario?

Answers

Multiple choice questions

1. *The correct answer is D.* The duty of candour was introduced after the Francis Inquiry into failings in basic patient care were exposed at Mid Staffordshire Hospital, where many patients died as a result of poor care over some considerable time but staff failed to recognise problems and report issues appropriately.

2. *The correct answer is D.* The responsible person should be the employer or a senior dentist who has the overall task of ensuring that the complaints procedure of the workplace is followed correctly for every complaint received. The actual handling of the complaint can be delegated to another member of staff, as the complaints manager, but the responsible person must check that the correct procedure is followed.

3. *The correct answer is E.* Acknowledgement of receipt of a complaint must be made within a few working days to the complainant. A written report of the investigation into the complaint and the conclusions reached by the workplace must be sent by recorded delivery to the complainant once the investigation is completed.

4. *The correct answer is D.* Storing the records in a central complaints file allows easy access to the paperwork for any relevant incident and maintains a system of good 'housekeeping'. Although a reference to a complaint can be noted in the patient's records, the actual record of the complaint should not be stored within the patient's records. The storage time for complaints records should be in line with the records management policy of the workplace.

5. *The correct answer is C.* When the complainant is unhappy with the conclusion of the workplace's in-house investigation, they have the right to take the matter further and make a formal complaint. The workplace must then provide the necessary contact information for either the NHS commissioning body, the Dental Complaints Service (for private patients) or the Health Service Ombudsman.

6. *The correct answer is E.* With the best will in the world, mistakes happen from time to time. The most important point for all concerned is to learn lessons from the mistake – how it happened, why it happened, what particular events allowed it to happen at that time and so on. Analysing this information retrospectively should allow the team to work out how the incident can be prevented in the future.

7. *The correct answer is C.* Social media is available to everyone and is a relatively uncontrolled platform for making comments about anything, both good and bad. Comments are best given directly to the workplace or to the relevant regulator. The Care Quality Commission actively encourages patients (and their carers or guardians) to contact them about the care they receive from all health and social care providers and expects all dental workplaces to have opportunities in place for their service users to make comments directly to them – especially using patient satisfaction surveys and written feedback such as 'thank you' cards.

8. *The correct answer is E.* The GDC expects all complaints to be handled and investigated in a timely manner, and complainants should be notified of this when their complaint is first acknowledged. When timescales alter, such as if a defence organisation becomes involved in the matter, the complainant should be notified promptly of these alterations to be kept abreast of the situation.

9. *The correct answer is B.* The Commissioning body in any geographical area is the local area team responsible for the operational management of NHS services in that area (including dentistry). All are overseen by the NHS Commissioning Board, which in turn is overseen by the Department of Health.

10. *The correct answer is A.* An apology at the receipt of a complaint indicating the workplace is sorry the patient is unhappy or aggrieved about the service they have received is acceptable, but this cannot be seen as an admission of liability.

11. *The correct answer is A.* Acknowledgement of receipt of a complaint must be made to the complainant within a few working days of its receipt. They must then be kept informed of how the complaint will be dealt with, who will be involved in the investigation and the expected timescales involved in investigating and concluding the report.

12. *The correct answer is B.* The Consumer Rights Act 2015 covers the provision of services to customers, including the provision of dental treatment (services) to customers (patients). It applies when a complaint has been found to be valid.

13. *The correct answer is B.* Although written records must be kept of all complaints received and their investigations and results, the number of complaints received and/or resolved is not required to be on display to patients in the workplace. This information should be held in the complaints folder and must be accessible to regulators such as the Care Quality Commission.

14. *The correct answer is C.* Principle 5 covers patients' expectations of the dental workplace if they have to make a complaint. They expect to be taken seriously when they complain and expect matters to be investigated thoroughly by the workplace. They should also be given contact information for other organisations such as the GDC and Care Quality Commission if they wish to take the matter further.

Extended matching questions

1. *The correct answer is b).* The patient should be given information on the relevant body to whom he may make a formal complaint about the incident, the appropriate body being dependent on whether the workplace runs under the NHS or privately.

2. *The correct answer is f).* The complaints policy should state the name of the 'responsible person' who ensures that the complaints procedure is followed correctly (usually a senior dentist) and the name of the complaints manager who receives all complaints. The name of the complaints manager must be displayed in a patient-accessible area of the workplace.

3. *The correct answer is e).* A written report must be produced for the complainant stating the findings of the investigation into the complaint by the complaints manager, with the conclusion of the investigation stated as one of these three options. The report should be sent by recorded delivery to the complainant to ensure it is received.

4. *The correct answer is a).* The receipt of a complaint by the dental workplace should be acknowledged within a few working days, either in writing or by telephone and followed by a written acknowledgement.

5. *The correct answer is c).* The complaints manager must investigate the complaint thoroughly, by giving the patient the opportunity to describe what happened and ideally what was said during the incident. The member of staff should also have the chance to tell their version of events, either with or without the patient present.

2a Raising Concerns and Safeguarding

Multiple choice questions

1. The General Dental Council (GDC) Standards document states that patients expect the dental team to act promptly to protect their safety if there are concerns about the cleanliness of the dental workplace. Which one of the following options is the term used to describe this action?
   A Complaining
   B Raising concerns
   C Reporting untoward incidents
   D Safeguarding children
   E Safeguarding vulnerable adults

2. When there are concerns about the health, performance or behaviour of a dental professional, colleagues have a duty to raise concerns appropriately. Which one of the following options is not an example of performance by a dental professional that should raise concerns?
   A Not meeting expected standards
   B Putting employer's interests last
   C Putting patients at risk
   D Putting patient's interests last
   E Working outside scope of practice

3. There may be instances when it is clear that a concern needs to be raised but the dental professional is unsure of who to complain to, for fear of being branded a troublemaker by the employer. Which one of the following options is the organisation to whom concerns about a colleague's fitness to practise should be made?
   A Care Quality Commission
   B Dental defence organisation
   C General Dental Council
   D Health and Safety Executive
   E Public Concern at Work

Questions and Answers for Dental Nurses, Fourth Edition. Carole Hollins.

4. All student dental nurses are required to work within a dental workplace during their training period so that they gain invaluable hands-on access to learning opportunities 'at the chairside'. Which one of the following options is the organisation that has a responsibility to report a patient safety issue involving a student?
   A Dental workplace
   B General Dental Council
   C National Examining Board for Dental Nurses
   D Public Concern at Work
   E Training course provider

5. In the interests of public safety, all people are encouraged to raise concerns about their workplace without fear of retribution from their employers. Which one of the following options is the legislation that protects whistle-blowers from vindictive dismissal by their employer?
   A Data Protection Act 1998
   B Freedom of Information Act 2000
   C Health and Safety at Work Act 1974
   D Public Interest Disclosure Act 1998
   E Reporting of Injuries, Diseases and Dangerous Occurrences Regulations 2013

6. Untoward incidents are those that occur unexpectedly and with unfavourable outcomes, such as a patient or staff member coming to harm while in the dental workplace. Which one of the following options is not classed as an untoward incident in the dental workplace?
   A Compressor failure
   B Disease transmission
   C Exposure to hazardous substance
   D Patient misidentification
   E Wrong site surgery

7. Any incident that has had an impact on patient safety, or had the potential to do so, should be reported to a central body for analysis and identification of common risks and system failures. Which one of the following options is the term used to describe incidents that had the potential to impact patient safety?
   A Accident
   B Complaint
   C Near miss
   D Safeguarding
   E Serious untoward incident

8. When an incident occurs in the dental workplace that results in a patient receiving serious injury or requires medical treatment to avoid serious injury or death,

the relevant national quality standards body must be notified immediately. Which one of the following options is the representation of the national quality standards bodies for Wales and Northern Ireland, respectively?

A CQC and HIW
B HIS and HIW
C HIS and RQIA
D HIW and RQIA
E RQIA and CQC

9. Chance and human error may play a part in an incident and can never be fully eliminated, but most safety incidents in the workplace occur because of systemic and recurrent failings that have not been identified and acted upon previously. Which one of the following options is the term used to describe the process that should be carried out to help reduce the occurrence of safety incidents in the workplace?

A Audit
B Policy formulation
C Risk assessment
D Satisfaction survey
E Standard operating procedures

10. Very occasionally the dental team may treat patients who are classed as vulnerable adults and who require the protection of their welfare and assurance of their safety from others. Which one of the following options is the term used to describe the actions required to achieve this?

A Prevention
B Raising concerns
C Reporting incidents
D Safeguarding
E Whistle-blowing

11. The General Dental Council (GDC) Standards document states that patients expect the dental team to act promptly to protect their safety if there are concerns about the clinical performance of a team member. Which one of the following options is the term used to describe this action?

A Complaining
B Raising concerns
C Reporting untoward incidents
D Safeguarding children
E Safeguarding vulnerable adults

12. There may be instances when it is clear that a concern needs to be raised but the dental professional is unsure of who to complain to, for fear of being branded a troublemaker by the employer. Which one of the following options

is the organisation to whom concerns about the workplace environment should be made?

A Care Quality Commission
B Dental defence organisation
C General Dental Council
D Health and Safety Executive
E Public Concern at Work

13. Once a concern has been raised in the dental workplace, it must be taken seriously and investigated promptly, in line with the underperformance and whistle-blowing policy of the workplace. Which one of the following options is an instance when a concern cannot be investigated in the workplace?

A Gagging clause in place
B Involves a minor issue
C Involves the employer
D No staff support system in place
E Self-employed staff involved

14. Children and vulnerable adults should be protected from harm and have others able to make decisions and allow interventions on their behalf, as they are deemed unable to do so themselves, especially in their own best interests. Which one of the following options is the legislation that stipulates this?

A Access to Health Records 1990
B Freedom of information Act 2000
C Health and Safety (Young Persons) Regulations 1997
D Mental Capacity Act 2005
E Public Interest Disclosure Act 1998

15. When a child or vulnerable adult is dependent on another person for their care and well-being, safeguarding issues may arise because that person has control over the child or vulnerable adult and their situation on a daily basis. Which one of the following options is the term used to describe a persistent failure by that person to meet the child or vulnerable adult's basic physical and/or psychological needs?

A Abuse of trust
B Emotional abuse
C Financial abuse
D Neglect
E Physical abuse

16. No member of the dental team would be expected to make a diagnosis of abuse, but all would be expected to recognise potential causes for concern and seek advice or report matters appropriately. Which one of the following options should be the first action to take by a dental team member who suspects their patient is the potential victim of abuse?

A Ask their escort to explain the injuries
B Contact the Care Quality Commission

C Contact the local Safeguarding Team
D Document any concerns and injuries present
E Phone the police

17. It is a requirement for all dental team members who have any contact with children or vulnerable adults to undergo an enhanced criminal records check, if they wish to continue to work in any of the dental care professions. Which one of the following options is the organisation tasked with carrying out these checks?
A Care Quality Commission (or national equivalent)
B Criminal Investigation Department
C Disclosure and Barring Service
D Local Safeguarding Board
E NHS Local Area Team

Extended matching questions

Topic: I

For each of the following raising concerns questions, select the single most appropriate answer from the option list. Each option might be used once, more than once or not at all.

a) General Dental Council
b) Health and Safety Executive
c) National Reporting and Learning System
d) Near miss
e) Public Concern at Work
f) Raising concerns
g) Risk assessment
h) Root cause analysis
i) Untoward incident
j) Whistle-blowing

1. For several months the senior dentist has noticed that the cash takings from patients for their dental treatment is short by around £40 each week, so decides to investigate the matter. The serial numbers of the bank notes in the cash box are recorded and at the end of a day when the takings are short again, all staff are requested to allow their own bank notes to be checked by the employer. An associate dentist is found to have the recorded notes in his possession. Which one of the options listed is the organisation to whom the incident should be reported by the employer?

2. A young dental nurse has been working in a dental workplace for several months when the vacuum autoclave breaks down and is out of use until an engineer can attend to repair it. In the meantime, staff are instructed to use the

downward displacement autoclave for all items, including the implant kits used by her employer. From her training, the nurse remembers that these items should be sterilised in a vacuum autoclave only and is concerned about the possibility of a cross-infection incident occurring, but she is unsure who to approach for advice as all her colleagues are following the employer's instructions. Which one of the options listed is an organisation concerned with advising people about compliance and malpractice issues such as this?

3. A staff meeting has been called following a patient safety incident in the workplace, where a patient slipped on a wet floor and broke his arm. The meeting aims to analyse the incident and determine the chain of events that led up to it happening, in an effort to prevent a similar incident in the future. Which one of the options listed is the correct term for this procedure?

Topic: II

For each of the following questions about safeguarding, select the requested number of most appropriate answers from the option list. Each option might be used once, more than once or not at all.

a) Abuse of trust
b) Care Quality Commission
c) Emotional abuse
d) Local Safeguarding Adult Board
e) Local Safeguarding Children Board
f) Neglect
g) Physical abuse
h) Police
i) Sexual abuse
j) Social services

1. A mother has attended with her 7-year-old daughter as an emergency patient, complaining that she has been awake all night with toothache. On examination, the dentist sees several deciduous teeth have gross caries and the lower left first permanent molar has a buccal swelling present. On checking the patient's records it seems four previous treatment appointments have been missed, and when questioned, the mother says she could not take time off work to attend. Which one of the options listed is the type of abuse that the mother is inflicting on her daughter in this scenario?

2. A husband and wife have attended for their dental examinations, and the dentist has noticed a deterioration in the husband's mental capacity – he seems unsure of why he is at the practice and how he arrived there. The dentist also

notices the husband has several scratches on his face and neck, and several old bruises on his forearms. The dentist suspects the husband is being physically abused by his wife or another person, and after discussing the issue with his dental defence organisation, he is advised to report the matter. Which two of the options listed are the bodies to whom the matter should be reported?

3. A young patient has attended with his father after apparently falling off his bike, but the dentist notices that the child has bilateral injuries to his cheeks and ears and soft tissue injuries to the inside of his lower lip. When the dentist asks the patient how he fell off his bike, the father butts in and prevents the child from answering. Which one of the options listed is the type of abuse that the dentist suspects the child is suffering?

4. A young student dental nurse has been placed in a training practice to complete the practical side of her nurse training but is uncomfortable with aspects of the workplace. One of the male associates she works with has asked her several times to join him for drinks after work, implying that if she does not he may be unable to sign off her Record of Experience document. Which one of the options listed is the type of abuse that the young student dental nurse is being exposed to?

Answers

Multiple choice questions

1. *The correct answer is C.* Any issue about the dental workplace that may affect the safety of patients while on the premises should be brought to the attention of the appropriate body accordingly. An unclean environment is likely to raise issues around infection prevention and control.

2. *The correct answer is B.* A dental professional's duty to raise a concern must override any personal and professional loyalty to the colleague causing the concern, including an employer.

3. *The correct answer is C.* The General Dental Council is the regulatory body of the whole dental profession, and all dental professionals are required to be registered annually with this organisation to work within their professional category.

4. *The correct answer is E.* Until student dental nurses pass their qualification examinations and enter the General Dental Council's register, their 'fitness to practise' is under the scrutiny of their training course provider. Any patient safety issues that occur during their training, such as drug abuse or failure to follow health and safety procedures, must be reported by the training provider to the General Dental Council and, if serious enough, may result in students losing their training place.

5. *The correct answer is D.* The Public Interest Disclosure Act is aimed at encouraging people to raise concerns about potentially dangerous or illegal practices in their workplace without fear of retribution from their employer. The General Dental Council's Standards document also states that employment contracts containing 'gagging' clauses should also be discouraged, for the same reason.

6. *The correct answer is A.* The failure of the compressor to work correctly is a routine, although irritating, event in the dental workplace and is likely to require the rescheduling of treatment sessions for patients once the machine is repaired. Regular servicing and maintenance of the compressor by a qualified engineer should reduce these instances considerably. Explosion of the compressor would be an untoward incident, however, and should be reported accordingly.

7. *The correct answer is C.* Near misses are effectively untoward incidents that were narrowly avoided, such as a patient about to receive a dose of penicillin having the medical history cross-checked and the prescriber realising that the patient has a penicillin allergy.

8. *The correct answer is D.* Health Inspectorate Wales (HIW) and the Regulation Quality Improvement Authority (RQIA) are the Welsh and Northern Irish equivalents of the Care Quality Commission (CQC) of England. Healthcare Improvement Scotland (HIS) is the Scottish quality standard body.

9. *The correct answer is C.* Risk assessments are a key element of identifying hazards in the workplace and determining how they can be reduced or ideally eliminated, so that the potential for anyone to suffer harm on the premises during a safety incident is minimal.

10. *The correct answer is D.* Safeguarding is the term used to describe the actions required by the dental team to protect a vulnerable adult (or child) from abuse or neglect by another person. Those who require safeguarding are deemed so because they may lack the mental capacity (either temporarily or permanently) to make decisions for themselves, especially decisions in their own best interest.

11. *The correct answer is B.* Raising a concern is not the same as making a complaint about an individual. The former does not require proof of malpractice, instead it highlights an issue that others (such as the GDC) should look into to determine if a problem exists.

12. *The correct answer is D.* Issues concerning an unsafe work environment where both staff and patients may come to harm should be reported to the Health and Safety Executive (HSE), as they are the organisation that determines how work environments can run safely. Any work-related injuries, diseases or dangerous occurrences that actually do happen on the premises must be reported to HSE under RIDDOR – this is a statutory requirement.

13. *The correct answer is C.* When the employer itself is the cause for concern, the matter may not be investigated thoroughly if at all or may be covered up by the employer. In these instances the complainant should seek advice elsewhere and, depending on the cause of the concern, this may be from Public Concern at Work, General Dental Council, Health and Safety Executive, etc.

14. *The correct answer is D.* The Mental Capacity Act expects that adults have the ability to make informed choices about themselves, their health and treatment and their care, while vulnerable adults and children may not have that ability. However, note the word 'may' – the Act also says that all adults should be assumed to have mental capacity until proved otherwise.

15. *The correct answer is D.* Failure to provide adequate food, clothing or shelter, or failure to supervise the vulnerable adult or child sufficiently so that they come into harm's way, or failure to ensure they receive prompt and effective medical or dental care when required are all examples of neglect.

16. *The correct answer is D.* Having a written record of their concerns and details of any injuries present forms evidence taken at the time. If the patient then presents with similar or further issues or injuries, the evidence can be collated and can help to make the decision whether to contact others for advice and help, such as the local Safeguarding Team.

17. *The correct answer is C.* The enhanced checks carried out by the Disclosure and Barring Service (DBS) are particularly thorough and should disclose convictions, police cautions and information on police investigations where a conviction or caution was not issued. DBS considers all adult patients are

vulnerable whilst undergoing dental treatment (rather than just those declared so under the Mental Capacity Act stipulations), so no one is exempt from their scrutiny during a DBS check.

Extended matching questions

Topic: I

1. *The correct answer is a).* The scenario describes an incident of theft, and the alleged thief is a registered dental professional with the General Dental Council (GDC). The GDC will investigate the matter as a 'fitness to practise' issue and may declare the associate to be guilty of serious professional misconduct. The incident should also be reported to the police.
2. *The correct answer is e).* Public Concern at Work is an independent authority that deals with whistle-blowing issues that are in the public interest, such as this. They encourage workers to raise concerns about malpractice and poor standards in their workplace and will guide them to report incidents to other organisations as necessary.
3. *The correct answer is h).* A root cause analysis is less about finding who to blame for an untoward incident and more about how the event occurred and why something went wrong. Changes can then be made to procedures for future incident prevention and feedback given to all staff about patient safety policy updates. A risk assessment is carried out before any events occur, in an effort to prevent them from happening.

Topic: II

1. *The correct answer is f).* The child is dependent on her mother for her care and well-being, as she is too young to attend the practice on her own. The mother is persistently failing to meet her daughter's basic physical need to have dental treatment and resolve her dental pain. This is neglect.
2. *The correct answers are d) and h).* Where abuse of a vulnerable adult is likely, both bodies should be contacted so the matter can be investigated thoroughly and the vulnerable adult removed from the unsafe environment for protection. All dental workplaces should hold contact information for their Local Safeguarding Boards for both vulnerable adults and children.
3. *The correct answer is g).* Accidental injuries tend to occur on one side of the body and affect bony prominences such as the knee or elbow. Unless the child went head first over the handlebars, the injuries described are unlikely to have occurred in a bike accident as they are bilateral. The actions of the father in preventing the child from speaking should also raise alarm in the dental team.
4. *The correct answer is a).* Th associate is in a position of power over the student and is using it to coerce her into doing something she does not wish to do, namely to have a social relationship with him. The student should report the issue immediately to her training course provider, who should report the matter to the senior dentist and remove the student from the workplace if necessary.

3 Oral Health Instruction

Multiple choice questions

1. Patient education about the various dental diseases, their causes, risk factors and prevention are of great importance in reducing the potential damage that these diseases may cause in the patient's mouth. The success of any patient education delivered by the dental team depends on various factors. Which one of the following options is the only factor that is under the dental team's control when delivering oral health education to a patient?
   A Age
   B Communication
   C General health
   D Mental capacity
   E Motivation

2. The prevention and control of dental caries, gingivitis and periodontitis revolves around educating patients in how each disease occurs initially, before determining their individual risk factors and how to change them. Which one of the following options is the patient's most important method of preventing both dental caries and gingivitis?
   A Change lifestyle
   B Control plaque
   C Fluoride application
   D Have regular scales
   E Reduce free sugars

3. Dental plaque biofilm consists of saliva, oral debris and mouth bacteria as a sticky layer that coats teeth and their gingival margins. When mouth bacteria ingest available food debris and produce weak acids, the pH level of the oral cavity is altered. Which one of the following options is the pH level at which these weak acids can start to cause enamel demineralisation?
   A pH 1.5
   B pH 3.5

Questions and Answers for Dental Nurses, Fourth Edition. Carole Hollins.

C pH 5.5
D pH 7.5
E pH 9.5

4. The dental team should use oral hygiene instruction sessions to recommend various oral health products to their patients, according to their needs. Which one of the following options is a product constituent that is usually recommended to patients suffering from dental sensitivity, especially to cold stimulation?
   A Arginine
   B Chlorhexidine
   C Hydrogen peroxide
   D Sodium fluoride
   E Triclosan

5. Controlling bacterial plaque daily is the main method by which patients can promote their own oral health, and the dental team can assist by advising on the various methods of plaque removal available. Which one of the following options is the usual method of removing bacterial plaque from the labial and buccal surfaces of the teeth?
   A Flossing
   B Interdental brushing
   C Mouth washing
   D Scaling
   E Toothbrushing

6. Toothbrushing is the commonest method of bacterial plaque removal carried out by the majority of patients, using either good-quality manual brushes or rechargeable electric brushes. Which one of the following options is advice about toothbrushing that should not be given to patients when offering oral hygiene instruction to them?
   A Brush for 2 minutes minimum
   B Brush twice daily minimum
   C Change brush when bristles deform
   D Press hard to contact teeth
   E Spit out but do not rinse

7. The interdental spaces are those lying between the mesial surface of one tooth and the distal surface of the adjacent tooth, just above the gingivae. The point where the two adjacent teeth touch together is the contact point, so interdental spaces vary in size from patient to patient dependent on whether their teeth are spaced out, just in contact or crowded together. Which one of the following options is usually the most effective method of bacterial plaque removal in an average interdental space?
   A Dental floss
   B Dental tape

C Interdental brush
D Interspace brush
E Toothpick

8. A wide range of mouthwashes are available for patient use ranging from shops' own brands to specialised products from oral health product suppliers. Like toothpastes, many mouthwashes contain specific ingredients for certain dental problems, such as sensitivity or periodontal disease. Which one of the following options is correct advice in relation to the regular use of a mouthwash as part of the patient's oral health regime?
   A Dilute for use
   B Swallow the solution
   C Use 30 minutes after brushing
   D Use immediately after brushing
   E Use instead of brushing

9. There are times when it is not possible to clean the teeth until several hours after a meal, such as when patients are at work or dining out. In these situations, they are advised to eat a 'detergent food' at the end of the meal to help stimulate saliva flow and remove at least some food debris from around and between the teeth. Which one of the following options is a good example of a 'detergent food'?
   A Apple
   B Cheesecake
   C Hard cheese
   D Milky coffee
   E Orange segment

10. Sugar-free chewing gum is widely available and is a useful adjunct to adequate oral hygiene in some circumstances, such as when consuming food away from home on a regular basis. As with 'detergent foods', chewing the gum stimulates saliva flow and helps to wash away food debris from around and between the teeth. Which one of the following options is good advice to give to patients in relation to chewing gum?
   A Any chewing gum is acceptable for use
   B Chew before meal to stimulate saliva
   C Dispose of when flavour has gone
   D Less abrasion effect than brushing
   E Use throughout day

11. The interdental spaces are those lying between the mesial surface of one tooth and the distal surface of the adjacent tooth, just above the gingivae. The point where the two adjacent teeth touch together is the contact point, so interdental spaces vary in size from patient to patient dependent on whether their teeth are spaced out, just in contact or crowded together. Which one of the

following options is an oral health product that does not remove bacterial plaque from these areas?
A Dental tape
B Flossette
C Interdental brush
D Manual toothbrush
E Sonic toothbrush

12. Toothbrushing is the commonest method of bacterial plaque removal carried out by the majority of patients, using either good-quality manual brushes or rechargeable electric brushes. Which one of the following options is advice given about toothbrushing that helps ensure the patient brushes all of the tooth surfaces at each session?
A Brush for 2 minutes minimum
B Brush twice daily minimum
C Change brush when bristles deform
D Press hard to contact teeth
E Spit out but do not rinse

13. Controlling bacterial plaque daily is the main method by which patients can promote their own oral health, and the dental team can assist by advising on the various methods of plaque removal available. Which one of the following options is the usual method of rinsing loose debris from the teeth and soft tissues while applying certain chemicals to them as required, such as plaque suppressants?
A Flossing
B Interdental brushing
C Mouth washing
D Scaling
E Toothbrushing

14. The dental team should use oral hygiene instruction sessions to recommend various oral health products to their patients, according to their needs. Which one of the following options is a product constituent that is usually recommended to patients suffering from soft tissue inflammation, such as occurs with subacute pericoronitis around partially erupted third molars?
A Biological enzyme
B Chlorhexidine
C Hydrogen peroxide
D Sodium fluoride
E Triclosan

Extended matching questions

For each of the following oral health instruction questions, select the requested number of most appropriate answers from the option list. Each option might be used once, more than once or not at all.

a) Apply fluoride
b) Change lifestyle
c) Have regular scales
d) Improve oral hygiene
e) Reduce free sugars
f) Use dental tape
g) Use interdental brush
h) Use interspace brush
i) Use manual brush
j) Use mouthwash
k) Use woodstick

1. A young adult patient has attended the practice for advice about effective cleaning of his lower anterior teeth, which are crowded. He is considering having orthodontic treatment in the future to straighten them but in the meantime, he regularly finds food debris stuck between the incisors and struggles to remove it. Which two of the options listed are the most likely cleaning aids to be recommended to the patient to improve his cleaning in this area?

2. A regular teenage patient has attended for a routine examination after having upper and lower fixed appliances fitted at the local hospital the previous month. The girl normally has excellent oral hygiene but is struggling to clean effectively beneath the archwires of the braces, and plaque is present today. Which one of the options listed is the most likely method of oral cleaning to be recommended to the patient to clean this area more efficiently?

3. A middle-aged patient is concerned that despite her best efforts, she always presents for her annual dental examination with tartar built up around her lower incisor teeth. The dentist explains that due to a high mineral content in her saliva, the patient is likely to continue with this experience although she has a good standard of oral hygiene elsewhere. Which one of the options listed is the most likely method of controlling the tartar build-up for this patient?

4. A middle-aged patient has attended the practice for the extraction of a periodontally involved upper incisor tooth and is concerned when the dentist tells him that several other anterior teeth have bone loss due to periodontitis. He is warned that they may require extraction in the future too. The patient has no signs of gingival inflammation as he is a smoker and believed his oral hygiene was adequate because his gums do not bleed when brushing. Which one of the options listed is the most likely advice that the dentist may give to this patient to improve his oral health?

Answers

Multiple choice questions

1. *The correct answer is B.* All members of the dental team require good levels of communication skills to enable them to advise and instruct their patients adequately. The team can try to motivate patients to improve their efforts when delivering oral health information, but whether patients become motivated to do so or not is their own decision.

2. *The correct answer is B.* The presence of bacterial plaque in a patient's mouth and around the teeth and gingivae is necessary for the formation of both dental caries and gingivitis. Consequently, its regular and efficient removal by the patient when carrying out oral hygiene techniques is the best method of preventing both diseases. Lifestyle changes and regular scales to remove calculus and other oral debris will help to control gingivitis only, whereas fluoride application and less free sugar consumption will help to reduce the incidence of dental caries only.

3. *The correct answer is C.* pH 5.5 is referred to as the critical pH level, as this is the level of acidity required to begin enamel demineralisation in the mouth. pH levels above 5.5 are not acidic enough to allow tooth damage to occur.

4. *The correct answer is A.* Arginine incorporated into toothpastes and used on a regular basis by the patient has been shown to be effective at reducing dental sensitivity. It acts by sealing dentinal tubules so that the nerve fibrils lying within them are less stimulated by cold sensation such as occurs with cold foods and drinks or exposure to cold air while breathing through the mouth.

5. *The correct answer is E.* The physical contact of the toothbrush bristles on the flat surfaces of the teeth, such as the labial and buccal surfaces, mechanically dislodges food debris and bacterial plaque from these areas. Both manual and electric toothbrushes achieve this cleaning action, although some electric brushes help to clean interdentally too.

6. *The correct answer is D.* The majority of abrasion cavities seen by the dental team have been caused by patients brushing with too much force in a 'sawing' action over the years. Good-quality brushes, whether electric or manual, should clean the teeth effectively without having to apply a hard force; indeed some electric brushes have alarms or flashing lights incorporated so that patients are made aware that they are applying too much force while brushing.

7. *The correct answer is C.* Correctly sized interdental brushes are ideal for cleaning debris from the interdental space, and they will brush the mesial and distal surfaces of the adjacent teeth too. Floss and tape are best at removing debris caught at the contact point, while interspace brushes are designed for use between spaced teeth and around fixed orthodontic components. Toothpicks may dislodge trapped interdental debris in some instances but provide no tooth cleaning effect and are often the cause of gingival trauma.

8. *The correct answer is C.* The chemicals contained in the toothpaste require sufficient time to act on the teeth and gingivae before being washed away while using a mouthwash. Current recommendation is to wait for 30 minutes after toothbrushing before using a mouthwash.

9. *The correct answer is A.* Detergent foods are raw, firm, fibrous fruits or vegetables that require a lot of chewing before being swallowed. The chewing action dislodges food debris from the teeth and stimulates saliva flow, which also helps to dislodge debris and restore a balanced pH level in the mouth. Hard cheese has no detergent effect on the teeth but does stimulate saliva flow and helps to neutralise organic acids in the mouth.

10. *The correct answer is C.* The flavour of the gum should last around 10 minutes, and this is adequate time for it to act as a 'detergent food'. Excessive chewing after this point or if used throughout the day increases the risk of tooth attrition. Only sugar-free chewing gum should be recommended, and 'detergent foods' need to be used after a meal, not before.

11. *The correct answer is D.* The head of a manual toothbrush is too large to clean between the teeth in the interdental spaces of all patients except those with many teeth missing in both arches. The sonic toothbrush has a vibrating head of bristles when in use, which creates a sonic wave of toothpaste slurry that passes through the interdental spaces, cleaning as it goes.

12. *The correct answer is A.* When carried out correctly and effectively, it should take a minimum of 2 minutes to brush the flat surfaces of the teeth in both arches. Patients should be advised to brush methodically around their mouths so that no area is missed and follow the same routine each time. Uppers first or lowers first, left side first or right side first – whatever is their preference, but they must ensure to brush all buccal, labial, lingual, palatal and occlusal surfaces of their teeth at each brushing session.

13. *The correct answer is C.* Mouth washing is not an alternative to effective toothbrushing, as the liquid only removes loose debris from the teeth and soft tissues. It is a useful technique at applying various chemicals to the teeth and gingivae, however, and, when forcibly sucked through anterior interdental areas by the patient, it can achieve a level of interdental cleaning too.

14. *The correct answer is C.* Hydrogen peroxide mouthwashes release oxygen when rinsed around the oral cavity, making them fizz. The oxygen acts against anaerobic bacteria (those that thrive in low-oxygen environments) that are usually associated with soft tissue wounds. The fizziness of the mouthwash also helps to mechanically dislodge debris from wound sites.

Extended matching questions

1. *The correct answers are f) and g).* Dental tape is designed to remove food debris that has become lodged in the contact point areas between the teeth, while correctly sized interdental brushes are ideal for cleaning the interdental

area between the teeth. Either product (or both) should be recommended to the patient and a demonstration given of their correct use.

2. *The correct answer is g).* Interdental brushes are available in a range of sizes, and their ends can be bent at an angle to the handle to access difficult areas such as beneath an archwire. Interspace brushes can be used to clean around brackets but are unlikely to clean beneath the archwire as well as interdental brushes.

3. *The correct answer is c).* The patient only attends once per year and has an adequate oral hygiene regime for all her other teeth, so the issue is not one of ineffective cleaning at home. The patient could attend more frequently for scaling of this area while maintaining her annual examination regime.

4. *The correct answer is b).* The dental team should always offer smoking cessation advice to their patients, in an effort to improve both their oral and general health. Some patients will not be receptive to this advice until they realise that their habit is affecting their health, such as when tooth extraction becomes necessary. Advice to change their lifestyle at a time when patients can see the negative consequences of their habit is more likely to be followed than at a time when they believe they have good oral and general health.

3a Disease Prevention and Health Advice

Multiple choice questions

1. Dental caries, gingivitis and periodontitis are the three main dental diseases of concern to the dental team. Advice on preventing them and providing treatment when one or more diseases are present forms the bulk of the daily work of the team. Which one of the following options is a common requirement in the prevention of all three dental diseases?
   A Control bacterial plaque build-up
   B Control the host response to disease
   C Modify any contributory factors
   D Modify the diet
   E Strengthen teeth against acids

2. Research has shown that fluoride can be incorporated into and onto the structure of teeth by the replacement of hydroxyapatite crystals with fluorapatite crystals. Which one of the following options is the main benefit of this new crystalline structure to the teeth of the patient?
   A More resistant to acid damage
   B More resistant to sugar damage
   C Reduces need for brushing
   D Removes unsightly mottling
   E Whitens teeth

3. The majority of toothpastes available to patients contain various fluoride salts that are present to help them reduce their caries experience, when used regularly. Which one of the following options is the current recommended level of fluoride (in parts per million – ppm) in toothpastes for use by adult patients with a high caries risk?
   A 1 ppm
   B 800 ppm
   C 1450 ppm
   D 5000 pm
   E 22,600 ppm

Questions and Answers for Dental Nurses, Fourth Edition. Carole Hollins.

4. Public health surveys have consistently shown the benefit of water fluoridation by comparing the 'decayed, missing, filled' (dmf – primary teeth, DMF – secondary teeth) tooth counts of fluoridated and non-fluoridated populations. Which one of the following options shows the percentage reduction in caries incidence of dmf/DMF counts in fluoridated populations against those of non-fluoridated populations?
   A 10%
   B 25%
   C 35%
   D 50%
   E 70%

5. The dental team have various techniques available to them to help protect their patients' teeth from carious attack, as well as offering regular oral hygiene advice and providing instruction in oral hygiene techniques. Which one of the following options is a technique specifically used to help protect difficult-to-clean areas such as the proximal surfaces of teeth?
   A Disclosing
   B Fissure sealing
   C Fluoride varnish application
   D Hall technique
   E Water fluoridation

6. The majority of toothpastes available to patients contain various fluoride salts that are present to help them reduce their caries experience, when used regularly. Which one of the following options is the current recommended level of fluoride (in parts per million – ppm) in toothpastes for general use by patients over the age of 3 years?
   A 1 ppm
   B 800 ppm
   C 1450 ppm
   D 5000 pm
   E 22,600 ppm

7. Modification of the diet is one of the key elements of advice given by the dental team in their efforts to reduce the caries experience of their patients, although it has little effect on reducing gingivitis or periodontitis. Which one of the following options is the most important oral health message to be given to patients in relation to free sugars and acidic drinks?
   A Brush teeth after consuming
   B Mouth wash before consuming
   C Reduce between-meal frequency
   D Take after meals only
   E Take before meals only

8. The dental team have various techniques available to them to help protect their patients' teeth from carious attack, as well as offering regular oral hygiene advice and providing instruction in oral hygiene techniques. Which one of the following options is a technique specifically used to help protect natural stagnation areas such as occlusal pits from becoming carious?
   A Disclosing
   B Fissure sealing
   C Fluoride varnish application
   D Hall technique
   E Water fluoridation

9. When giving dietary advice to patients the dental team must make them aware of harmful foods and drinks that contain 'hidden sugars' – so called because they are added during manufacturing to food products that would not be considered as 'sugary', such as savoury marinades and tinned vegetables. Which one of the following options is an example of a food product containing 'hidden sugars'?
   A Chocolate bar
   B Mackerel fillets in tomato sauce
   C Natural yogurt
   D Pineapple chunks in natural juice
   E Salted crisps

10. The Food Standards Agency produced their 'Eatwell Guide' to help advise the public on what constitutes a healthy balanced diet, by dividing a standard food plate into thirds and indicating the amounts of food products that should come from each food group. Which one of the following options are food groups that should form two-thirds of the standard food plate?
   A Fats and starchy carbohydrates
   B Fruit and vegetables, sugars
   C Proteins and fats
   D Starchy carbohydrates, fruits and vegetables
   E Sugars, proteins and fats

11. Fluoride can be taken into the enamel structure by direct application onto the teeth (topical fluoride) or by being taken internally (systemic fluoride). Which one of the following options is an example of a systemic fluoride application technique?
   A Fluoride drops
   B Fluoride varnish
   C Impregnated floss
   D Mouthwash
   E Toothpaste

12. Research has revealed that there are many links between oral diseases such as periodontitis and general health issues such as type II diabetes and heart disease. Which one of the following options is a health link that the dental team are particularly well placed to deliver to their patients?
    A Dental caries and high cholesterol
    B Dental caries and obesity
    C Gingivitis and dementia
    D Gingivitis and heart attacks
    E Periodontitis and high cholesterol

13. In relation to existing periodontal disease, contributory factors are those that aggravate the disease so that its extent is worse than would otherwise have been the case. Which one of the following options is a recognised contributory factor of periodontitis that exacerbates the disease by altering the patient's ability to heal effectively after a pathogen attack?
    A Diabetes
    B Epilepsy
    C Heart failure
    D Hypertension
    E Radiotherapy treatment

14. Some patients are prone to develop periodontal disease due to their genetic make-up, no matter how good their oral hygiene is and often without any contributory factors either. These patients require regular help from the dental team to control the build-up of plaque and calculus in the mouth. Which one of the following options is a constituent of toothpaste that actively suppresses the build-up of dental plaque and calculus that could be recommended to these patients?
    A Biological enzyme
    B Hydrogen peroxide
    C Sodium fluoride
    D Stannous fluoride
    E Triclosan with zinc

15. The dietary and lifestyle advice given by the dental team to maintain good oral health is also relevant to maintaining good general health, as the risk factors for both are very similar. Which one of the following options is a risk factor linked to both periodontal disease and heart disease?
    A Bulimia
    B Diabetes
    C Epilepsy
    D Sjogren's syndrome
    E Smoking

16. Oral cancer is one of the few cancers with an increasing incidence in the UK, particularly among younger patients. The dental team are in an ideal position to recognise suspicious oral lesions and make early referrals as well as to give

relevant dietary and lifestyle advice to patients at risk. Which one of the following options is an area of dietary advice that is not relevant to oral cancer?

A Fats and red meats
B Free sugars
C Fresh fruit
D Green vegetables
E Vitamin A

Extended matching questions

For each of the following disease prevention and health advice questions, select the requested number of most appropriate answers from the option list. Each option might be used once, more than once or not at all.

a) 1450 ppm
b) 5000 ppm
c) 22,600 ppm
d) Crowded teeth
e) Hydrogen peroxide
f) Mouth breathing
g) Sodium fluoride
h) Stannous fluoride
i) Unbalanced occlusion

1. A university student has attended for his routine dental examination during the summer holidays and complains of suffering from dental sensitivity whenever he has cold drinks. The dentist can see that several of the student's anterior teeth have wear facets present and diagnoses that the patient is bruxing. Which one of the options listed is a toothpaste constituent that should help to relieve the sensitivity issues for the student, when used regularly?

2. A regular elderly patient to the practice has recently been diagnosed with Alzheimer's disease, and the dental team have already noticed a deterioration in his mental capacity. The patient has maintained his dentition well over the years and only has two teeth missing, so the team are keen to assist him in looking after them for the rest of his life. Which one of the options listed is the most likely concentration of fluoride toothpaste to be recommended for use by the patient, in an effort to provide a higher level of protection against caries?

3. A young adult patient attends the practice to ask for advice about tooth whitening ready for her wedding later that summer. On examination, the dentist notices that she has a good overall standard of oral hygiene but that she has labial gingivitis affecting her upper anterior teeth. Which one of the options listed is the most likely reason for this area to develop inflammation in the absence of poor oral hygiene?

Answers

Multiple choice questions

1. *The correct answer is A.* The presence of bacterial plaque is associated with the onset of dental caries when the plaque forms on the hard tissues of the tooth. When the plaque forms in the gingival crevice it is associated with the onset of gingivitis, and when it becomes attached to existing calculus and is able to form subgingivally it is associated with the progression to periodontitis.

2. *The correct answer is A.* Fluorapatite crystals chemically are a stronger crystalline structure than hydroxyapatite and are able to resist attack by acids more easily.

3. *The correct answer is D.* Specialist high-fluoride products such as 'Duraphat' toothpaste are recommended for patients with an existing high rate of caries or who are high caries risk patients. The products are particularly useful for adult patients with a limited ability to clean their teeth effectively due to physical or mental disability.

4. *The correct answer is D.* Repeated research into the benefits of water fluoridation to a population consistently shows a reduction in caries incidence of 50% in those areas benefitting from the service against those that do not.

5. *The correct answer is C.* The proximal surfaces of the teeth (mesial of one and distal of the adjacent tooth) are natural stagnation areas where food debris can easily collect. Regular fluoride varnish applications to these areas can reduce the incidence of caries in the patient by 30% to 40%.

6. *The correct answer is C.* Once over 3 years old, it is currently recommended that all patients use 'adult' strength toothpastes containing 1450 ppm fluoride to provide the maximum protection against caries. Younger children should be supervised by parents during toothbrushing sessions to ensure they do not use too large an amount or ingest the toothpaste.

7. *The correct answer is C.* Confining ingestion of these cariogenic and erosive foods and drinks to mealtimes only (so three times daily only), rather than between meals too, enables the excess saliva produced at mealtimes to naturally wash them away, thus reducing the risk of enamel damage. Brushing teeth after the consumption of acidic drinks will cause more enamel damage, and mouth washing before their consumption will have little effect on enamel protection.

8. *The correct answer is B.* Fissure sealing involves the use of either glass ionomer or flowable composite products to permanently cover over tooth fissures and pits so that they no longer act as stagnation areas on the teeth. When not fissure sealed, these areas are prone to becoming choked with food debris, which requires removing to avoid causing demineralisation.

9. *The correct answer is B.* Savoury products containing tomato sauce are notorious for having a hidden sugar content as it is believed to make the product more palatable. Natural products and plain salted crisps do not have hidden sugars added, and everyone is aware that a chocolate bar contains sugar.

10. *The correct answer is D.* The other third of the plate should in total be made up of proteins, dairy products (and alternatives), small amounts of unsaturated oils and fats and very small amounts of sugars.

11. *The correct answer is A.* Fluoride drops can be added to drinks or given as drops directly to the young patient. They are especially useful in areas where there is no artificial water fluoridation and no natural fluoride content in drinking water supplies. In areas where some water fluoridation exists, the amount of fluoride drops to be taken needs to be calculated by the dentist to ensure the patient does not receive too high a level.

12. *The correct answer is B.* The vast majority of food products and drinks that are capable of causing dental caries are products that are also associated with causing obesity, mainly because of their sugar content but also because many are processed or convenience foods, with some hidden sugars content too.

13. *The correct answer is A.* Diabetic patients are referred to as being immunocompromised, as the illness alters their ability to fight infection or heal effectively when attacked by pathogens. Type 1 (insulin dependent) diabetics tend to be more aware of this issue than type 2 diabetics, many of whom remain undiagnosed until an accident, medical emergency or illness results in suitable hospital tests being carried out.

14. *The correct answer is E.* Earlier toothpastes contained just triclosan as an antiseptic plaque suppressant, but research has shown that when combined with zinc, the plaque suppression and antiseptic properties are far greater.

15. *The correct answer is E.* Several of the products present in tobacco cause narrowing of blood vessels; this is why smokers with periodontal disease rarely suffer from bleeding gingivae and are therefore unaware they have a problem. Similarly, the tobacco products cause narrowing of the blood vessels supplying the heart so that its correct functioning is reduced and they develop heart disease.

16. *The correct answer is B.* Research into oral cancers (especially squamous cell carcinoma – SCC) has shown links between the disease and diets high in fats and red meats and low in vitamin A. Definite links have been established between SCC and diets low in fresh fruit and vegetables.

Extended matching questions

1. *The correct answer is h).* Stannous fluoride within the toothpaste will help to calm the thermal stimulation affecting the nerve fibrils of the pulp tissue within the dentine, so the cold sensitivity gradually settles down. Regular use of the toothpaste should prevent the problem from recurring.

2. *The correct answer is b).* High-concentration fluoride toothpastes are available (sometimes on prescription) for use by patients with special needs, such as medical or physical conditions that make them more likely to suffer from dental caries. Dementias (such as Alzheimer's disease) gradually reduce the patients' ability to look after themselves adequately, including carrying out regular and effective toothbrushing. The use of high-fluoride toothpaste helps to counteract the reducing level of oral care and the increased risk of developing carious lesions.

3. *The correct answer is f).* Some patients habitually breathe through their mouth rather than nose, while others have a short upper lip that often cannot form a complete oral seal. Others have a malocclusion that prevents them closing their mouth fully. Whichever the problem, breathing through the mouth on a regular basis causes unnatural drying of the upper labial gingiva and eventually results in inflammation of the area.

3b Pre- and Post-operative Advice

Multiple choice questions

1. Many dental procedures require patients to have a local anaesthetic administered before undergoing treatment so that they feel comfortable during the procedure. Which one of the following options is a sensation felt by the tooth that is not usually lost to the patient after receiving a local anaesthetic?
   A Cold
   B Hot
   C Pain
   D Pressure
   E Tenderness

2. Fixed orthodontic treatment is carried out on both teenage and adult patients to correct various malocclusions, but the brackets bonded to the teeth act as stagnation areas for food debris and plaque. Which one of the following options is the oral health aid most likely to be recommended for removal of this debris and plaque from around the brackets, after the appliance has been bonded?
   A Floss
   B Interspace brush
   C Manual toothbrush
   D Superfloss
   E Tape

3. When a patient undergoes an extraction procedure it is usual for them to be given post-operative advice by the dental team, to avoid any complications developing in the following 24 hours such as the onset of reactionary haemorrhage. Which one of the following options is an action that the patient does not need to avoid doing during this time frame, as it is unlikely to cause reactionary haemorrhage?
   A Drink alcohol
   B Drink hot beverages

Questions and Answers for Dental Nurses, Fourth Edition. Carole Hollins.

C Eat food
D Rinse the mouth
E Take exercise

4. Following an accident while playing rugby, a young patient has suffered an avulsion of his upper left central incisor tooth and his mother has phoned for advice about handling the tooth while they proceed to the practice. Which one of the following options is the most likely advice to be given in this situation if the tooth is to be re-implanted?
   A Brush with toothpaste
   B Immerse in milk
   C Pack in ice
   D Rinse with mouthwash
   E Wrap in cotton wool

5. Once a tooth has been restored successfully with composite material under local anaesthesia, the patient is given post-operative instructions that include the advice not to attempt to eat anything until the anaesthetic has worn off. Which one of the following options is the reason for this advice to be given to the patient?
   A Allows setting of the material
   B Avoids damage to the tooth
   C Avoids dislodging the restoration
   D Avoids soft tissue trauma
   E Avoids staining the restoration

6. Before a patient undergoes a tooth extraction, it is usual procedure for the dentist to take a periapical radiograph of the tooth after gaining consent from the patient to do so. Which one of the following options is the reason given to the patient for this radiograph to be taken?
   A Check for caries
   B Check for periapical pathology
   C Check for periodontal disease
   D Check for root curvature
   E Check the number of roots

7. When a patient is to undergo dental treatment under intravenous conscious sedation, an assessment appointment is carried out before the treatment day and written pre-operative and post-operative instructions are provided by the dental team. Which one of the following options is a pre-operative instruction that the patient should be given at the assessment appointment in relation to the treatment day?
   A Attend with an adult escort
   B Have cash for taxi fare home
   C Leave dentures out
   D Starve for 6 hours beforehand
   E Stop all medications beforehand

8. Sometimes a patient may experience a dental problem but be unable to indicate which tooth is the cause of the trouble. The dentist may then resort to carrying out a vitality test on several adjacent teeth to identify the problem tooth. Which one of the following options is the sensation the patient should be told to expect when using ethyl chloride during the vitality test?
   A Cold sensation
   B Hot sensation
   C No sensation
   D Pain sensation
   E Tingling sensation

9. Many patients perform parafunctional actions with their teeth, such as bruxing during stressful periods. This often results in face and jaw ache or a fractured tooth, so the dentist often recommends they wear a dental guard to alleviate the symptoms. Which one of the following options is an incorrect cleaning and maintenance instruction for a dental guard?
   A Clean with toothpaste after wearing
   B Immerse in mouthwash when not wearing
   C Keep away from heat sources
   D Store in box provided
   E Use hot water to clean

10. A dental bridge is a device used to replace one or more missing teeth in a patient's mouth and can be constructed in a variety of designs. One such design is a simple cantilever, where the abutment teeth are on one side only of the missing tooth/teeth. Which one of the following options is an oral hygiene product that is unlikely to be recommended for cleaning under the pontic of this type of bridge?
    A Dental floss
    B Dental tape
    C Manual toothbrush
    D Sonic toothbrush
    E Superfloss

11. A patient has had an acrylic denture made to replace several missing teeth and has asked for advice on how to clean it correctly. Which one of the following options is suitable cleaning advice for the denture?
    A Clean while wearing, with other teeth
    B Clean fitting surface
    C Should not need cleaning
    D Soak in mouthwash solution
    E Soak overnight in bleach solution

12. Endodontic treatment is usually carried out to avoid the extraction of a tooth that cannot be saved otherwise. The procedure may require several appointments to complete fully, and then the tooth is restored with a filling for a period of time to ensure the treatment has been successful. Which one of the

following options is further treatment that is likely to be recommended for the tooth to the patient by the dental team, once the tooth is asymptomatic?
A Bridge placement
B Crown placement
C Extraction
D Filling replacement
E Tooth whitening

13. An anxious patient requires a grossly carious tooth to be extracted but is unwilling to undergo the procedure without being provided with some form of anxiety relief by the dental team. His medical history update has revealed he suffers from cirrhosis of the liver. Which one of the following options is the most likely form of anxiety relief to be discussed with the patient before he attends the treatment session?
A Dual drug intravenous sedation
B General anaesthesia
C Inhalation sedation
D Oral sedation
E Single drug intravenous sedation

14. After undergoing an extraction procedure earlier in the day, a patient's wife has phoned the dental workplace to request advice as the socket has started bleeding again. Which one of the following options is correct advice to give in this situation?
A Begin hot salt-water mouthwashes
B Bite onto a cotton pad for 30 minutes
C Go to Accident & Emergency
D Rinse the mouth to remove the blood
E Squeeze the socket with fingers

Answers

Multiple choice questions

1. *The correct answer is D.* Pressure sensation, or proprioception, is supplied by nerves present in the surrounding gingivae and especially the periodontal ligament fibres. Once the tooth has been anaesthetised, some of these nerve fibres in the soft tissues will detect pressure, but not pain. Hence the reason why, during a tooth extraction, the patient is aware of the tooth being pushed and 'wiggled' but feels no pain and is able to allow the extraction to proceed.
2. *The correct answer is B.* Interspace brushes have a tuft of bristles rather than a full head of bristles and are ideal for cleaning tricky areas such as around orthodontic brackets. Manual toothbrush heads are too large to do so, while all other options cannot be used to clean around brackets.
3. *The correct answer is C.* The patient should be advised to eat once their numbness wears off, but to avoid the side of the mouth where the extraction occurred as far as possible. All other options are likely to cause reactionary haemorrhage if carried out and should be avoided in the first 24 hours.
4. *The correct answer is B.* Immersing the avulsed tooth in water would suffice in most instances, but where milk is available this should be used preferentially. The calcium content of the milk is believed to help the cementum cells to survive the avulsion more readily, keeping them alive so that they can re-form an attachment with the socket once the tooth is re-implanted.
5. *The correct answer is D.* Modern composite materials are set at the time of insertion using a curing light, so they do not require time to set, they cannot be dislodged once set and they should not take up stain. The tooth has been restored to return its chewing function, and this should not cause damage to the tooth. The soft tissues will remain numb until the anaesthetic wears off, and during this time they are vulnerable to being bitten by the patient while trying to eat and causing trauma without the patient feeling anything.
6. *The correct answer is D.* If the tooth is being extracted the presence of any disease or pathology is irrelevant. The presence of any root curvature will affect the ease or difficulty of the extraction and allows the dentist to be forewarned of any potential problems – if severe curvature is present, then a surgical approach can be planned for. The dentist should be aware of the likely number of roots present on any tooth, although third molars occasionally cause surprise.
7. *The correct answer is A.* Patients must have an adult escort available to see them safely home after the procedure as they will remain under the effects of the drug for some hours afterwards and are effectively a vulnerable adult. The patient must never be IV sedated unless a suitable escort is with them. None of the other options are relevant.

8. *The correct answer is A.* Ethyl chloride is a liquid that vaporises at room temperature, producing ice crystals as it does so. When these crystals are formed on a cotton wool roll which is then held against the tooth, a cold sensation should be felt.

9. *The correct answer is E.* The material used to form a dental guard will distort out of shape if it is exposed to hot water or other sources of heat such as a radiator or fire. Dental guards should be cleaned with toothpaste and cold water after wearing.

10. *The correct answer is C.* Floss, tape and Superfloss can all be passed under the pontic to clean its underside and the underlying gingiva. The sonic effect of the electric toothbrush will also pass into this area and clean it effectively, but a manual brush will be unable to clean the area as the bristles will not get under the pontic adequately.

11. *The correct answer is B.* The fitting surface is that which is in contact with the soft tissues of the roof of the mouth and is the likeliest area for micro-organisms to attach to the denture and proliferate, especially fungi. This area should be cleaned every day with a soft brush and toothpaste or denture paste and therefore needs to be removed from the mouth to do so. The patient's own teeth should be cleaned too, while the denture is out. Soaking in mouthwash is insufficient for removing debris and micro-organisms, and bleach solution will gradually harden the acrylic and change its colour.

12. *The correct answer is B.* Root filled teeth are dead and tend to become brittle with time, so they require full cuspal protection once the tooth has fully settled. This is achieved by placing a crown on the tooth.

13. *The correct answer is C.* Inhalation sedation involves the use of a mixture of oxygen and nitrous oxide gases to be breathed in by the patient to produce an adequate level of anxiety relief. The nitrous oxide is not absorbed into the body, it is just exhaled out again so the liver is not involved in detoxifying the gas to remove it from the body. All other options involve the liver being able to detoxify the sedative drugs and when cirrhosis is present, the liver may be too diseased to do so.

14. *The correct answer is B.* Rinsing the mouth will remove any remaining blood clot and cause further bleeding still, while squeezing the socket with the fingers is likely to introduce infection to the area. The patient should be seen at the practice rather than at Accident & Emergency. Biting onto a cotton pad for 30 minutes should be sufficient to squash the blood vessels around the socket and stop the bleeding again as a clot re-forms.

Development Outcome B: Management and Leadership

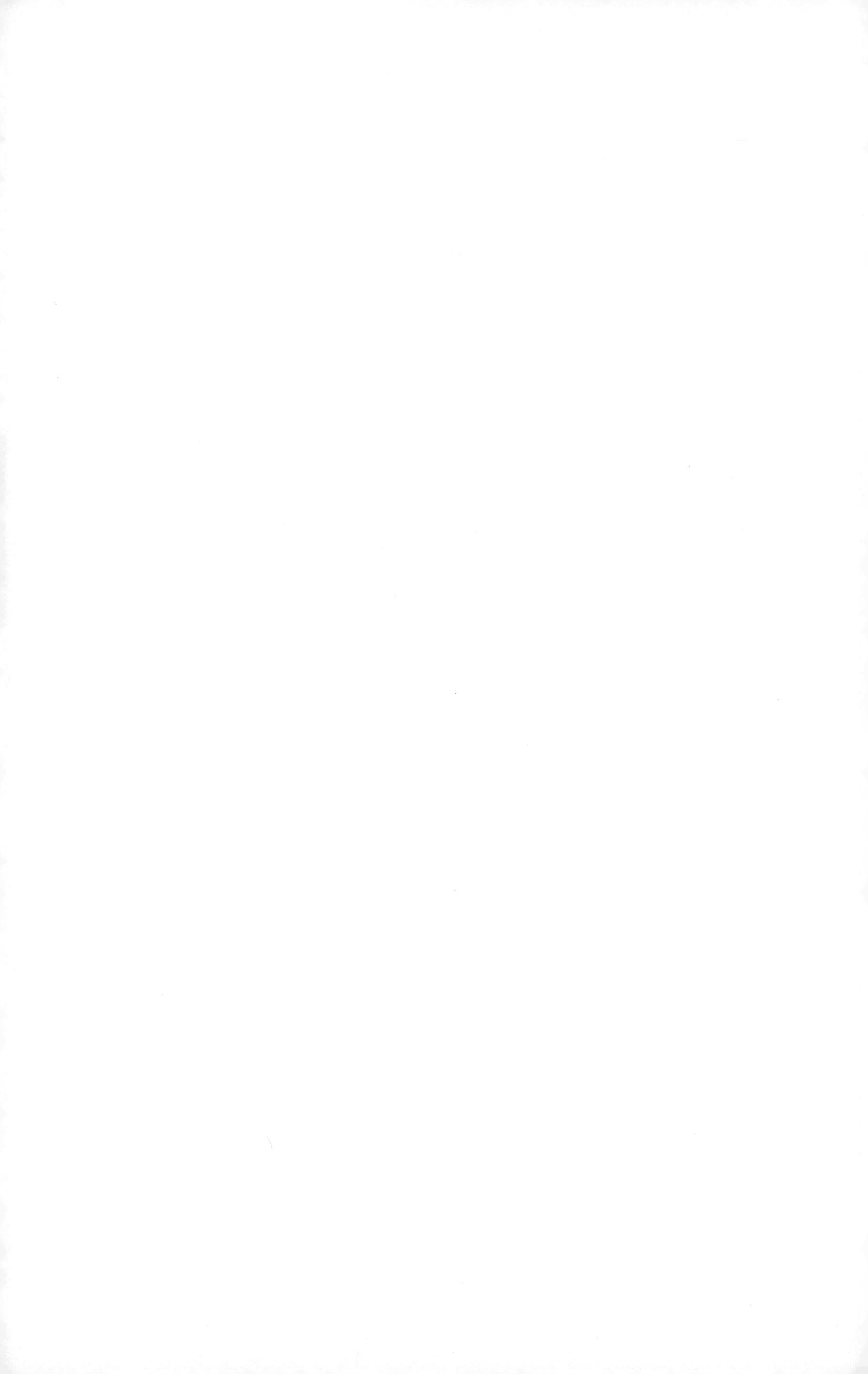

4 Teamwork and Chairside Support

Multiple choice questions

1. A large part of a dental nurse's time is involved with providing chairside assistance to clinical colleagues, whether they are dentists, therapists or hygienists. This involves having the clinical area correctly prepared before a treatment session and also assisting during treatment as necessary. Which one of the following options is a list of actions that should be carried out by the dental nurse at the end of a treatment day?
   A Empty bins, empty water bottle, switch off X-ray machine
   B Leave instruments in soak, empty bins, switch off computer
   C Reprocess instruments, switch off X-ray machine, wipe down surfaces
   D Switch off equipment, empty bins, leave instruments in soak
   E Wipe down surfaces, empty bins, reprocess instruments

2. Good teamwork involves several people working together safely and in harmony so that the end result of their actions is greater and more productive than if they each worked alone. Which one of the following options is an example of ineffective teamwork in the dental workplace?
   A Avoiding discrimination
   B Delegating effectively
   C Giving financial bonus selectively
   D Informing patient of team members' role in their care
   E Referring effectively

3. A large part of a dental nurse's time is involved with providing chairside assistance to clinical colleagues, whether they are dentists, therapists or hygienists. With dentists, one of the nurse's duties is to accurately record the dictated clinical findings during an oral health assessment appointment. Which one of the following options is information that is recorded in relation to a patient's need for orthodontic treatment to be carried out?
   A Alphanumeric charting
   B BPE score

Questions and Answers for Dental Nurses, Fourth Edition. Carole Hollins.

C FDI charting
D IOTN score
E PAR score

4. The dental team consists of several categories of registrant, each with a list of duties that they can perform that their relevant qualification entitles them to carry out. During their training they will have received the knowledge, skills and experience to do so. Which one of the following options is the specific General Dental Council publication that provides information to registrants on this issue?
   A *Enhanced CPD Guidance*
   B *Preparing for Practice*
   C *Scope of Practice*
   D *Standards for the Dental Team*
   E *Student Professionalism and Fitness to Practise*

5. Within the dental team registrants will have achieved various qualifications; from basic through extended to post-registration and post-graduate levels. This results in a wide range of skills and experience in the dental workplace. Which one of the following options is not a beneficial outcome of this ability range within the dental workplace?
   A Allows delegation of less complex duties
   B Dentist can work alone
   C Higher skilled carry out more complex duties
   D More patients treated effectively
   E Work time used more efficiently

6. A large part of a dental nurse's time is involved with providing chairside assistance to clinical colleagues, whether they are dentists, therapists or hygienists. This involves having the clinical area correctly prepared before a treatment session and also assisting during treatment as necessary. Which one of the following options is a list of actions that should be carried out by the dental nurse between each patient during a treatment session?
   A Change water bottle, dispose of PPE, switch on X-ray machine
   B Dispose of PPE, wipe instruments for re-use, change water bottle
   C Remove used instruments for processing, empty bins, wipe down chair
   D Switch off X-ray machine, wipe down surfaces, empty water bottle
   E Wipe down surfaces, dispose of waste items, remove used instruments for processing

7. Effective delegation involves a patient receiving simpler treatment from a suitably trained team member while only more complex treatment is carried out by more highly qualified colleagues. This makes the best use of all team members' time and skills during the working day. Which one of the following options is an example of effective delegation in the dental workplace?
   A Dental nurse sending appointment reminder
   B Dentist taking patient payment
   C Hygienist checking stock items

D Receptionist booking patient appointment
E Therapist decontaminating instruments

8. A large part of a dental nurse's time is involved with providing chairside assistance to clinical colleagues, whether they are dentists, therapists or hygienists. Which one of the following options is an area of chairside assisting that involves the dental nurse adequately removing fluids and debris from the patient's mouth during treatment?
   A Aspirating
   B Chaperoning
   C Decontaminating
   D Record keeping
   E Retracting

9. The General Dental Council's publication *Scope of Practice* identifies the skill levels expected of each registrant group upon their respective qualification in their chosen profession. Dental nurses may then carry out extended duties within the dental workplace in certain circumstances. Which one of the following options is an acceptable circumstance for extended duties to be carried out by a dental nurse?
   A During a dental emergency
   B During a staff shortage period
   C Following competency training
   D Following delegation by a team member
   E When instructed by the employer

10. Good teamwork involves several people working together safely and in harmony so that the end result of their actions is greater and more productive than if they each worked alone. Which one of the following options is an example of ineffective teamwork in the dental workplace?
   A Avoiding bullying or harassment
   B Delegating to team members
   C Non-registrant advising on dental care
   D Respecting individual roles
   E Treating all team members with respect

11. A large part of a dental nurse's time is involved with providing chairside assistance to clinical colleagues, whether they are dentists, therapists or hygienists. With dentists, one of the nurse's duties is to accurately record the dictated clinical findings during an oral health assessment appointment. Which one of the following options is information that is recorded in relation to the health of the gingival tissues?
   A Alphanumeric charting
   B BPE score
   C FDI charting
   D IOTN score
   E PAR score

12. Wherever possible all registrants should be appropriately supported by another team member while providing treatment to a patient, not only for the safety of the patient but also to act as a chaperone. Which one of the following options is an accepted circumstance where a registrant may provide care to a patient without a second team member being present?
    A Carrying out simple restorative procedure
    B Holiday periods
    C Out-of-hours emergency
    D Short-staffed periods
    E When treating adult patients

13. A large part of a dental nurse's time is involved with providing chairside assistance to clinical colleagues, whether they are dentists, therapists or hygienists. This involves having the clinical area correctly prepared before a treatment session and also assisting during treatment as necessary. Which one of the following options is a list of actions that should be carried out at the start of each treatment day by the dental nurse?
    A Check day list, clean instruments, set up local syringes
    B Collect instruments, set up local syringes, run DUWLs
    C Collect laboratory items, run DUWLs, check day list
    D Run DUWLs, check day list, switch on X-ray machine
    E Switch on X-ray machine, collect laboratory items, clean instruments

Answers

Multiple choice questions

1. *The correct answer is E.* The X-ray machine should only be switched on when its use is imminent and not left on otherwise. Instruments must be reprocessed at the end of the day and ready for use for the next day, not left in soak overnight. All surfaces must be wiped down and the bins emptied at the end of the day, with fresh orange sacks being placed ready for the next day.
2. *The correct answer is C.* When the dental workplace runs smoothly and effectively so that patients are treated to a high standard and in a timely manner, it usually happens due to good teamwork and everyone pulling together for the good of the patients. If only some members of the team are then rewarded by receiving a bonus while others are not, an air of resentment will develop – an 'us and them' split amongst team members that is likely to be destructive to the business and therefore to patient care.
3. *The correct answer is D.* The index of orthodontic treatment needs (IOTN) is a system used to grade a malocclusion or other orthodontic issue (such as crowding, tooth impaction or hypodontia) to determine whether the patient requires orthodontic intervention or not. Currently, only the most severe cases are likely to receive treatment under the NHS.
4. *The correct answer is C.* The *Scope of Practice* document describes the duties applicable to each category of registrant – what they have been trained to do during their training course and are deemed competent to do once they achieve their qualification. This allows various members of the team to have various duties delegated to them by more senior registrants in the team, so that the most highly qualified carry out the more complex duties while other team members can provide more routine levels of care.
5. *The correct answer is B.* Dentists should never work alone, without another team member to assist them and act as a chaperone, except when providing out-of-hours emergency care if necessary. All other options are beneficial outcomes of having a multi-talented team.
6. *The correct answer is E.* The water bottle is normally emptied at the end of each day and should not need changing beforehand. Likewise, the bins are normally emptied at the end of each day or each clinical session if necessary. Surfaces must be wiped down between patients and waste items must be disposed of then too. Used instruments must be removed from the clinical area to the decontamination room after each patient.
7. *The correct answer is D.* One of the duties of the reception staff is to book patient appointments. All other options are examples of higher-qualified staff carrying out duties that should be delegated to lesser-qualified staff – each option is an example of inefficiency.

8. *The correct answer is A.* The aspirator unit has high-speed and low-speed suction devices attached, the former for use while handpieces or scaler units are in use and the latter to remove saliva without the patient constantly swallowing while restorations are being placed. The dental nurse operates either system as required.

9. *The correct answer is C.* The various extended duties available to dental nurses can only be carried out once they have received suitable training to do so. This does not need to be formal training with an examination at the end of it. It can be carried out in-house by a more senior member of the team, but there must be a period of training given, recorded as being given, and the senior colleague must decide the colleague is competent in the duty before allowing them to provide care to patients.

10. *The correct answer is C.* If team members are non-registrants (such as some reception or administration staff, or students), they have not received the training to enable them to advise on dental care. Their only knowledge of such information is likely to be from personal experience or from listening to registrant colleagues advising patients.

11. *The correct answer is B.* A basic periodontal examination (BPE) should be carried out on adults at each oral health assessment appointment. It is used to quickly record the gingival health of the patient and identify areas where problems are present or are at risk of developing.

12. *The correct answer is C.* The dentist is responsible for providing emergency out-of-hours care and cannot expect staff members to be available to assist. The dentist must risk assess the situation and determine whether it is safe to provide treatment in each circumstance. Temporary treatments and simple treatments may be safely provided while working alone, but other treatments should be delayed until normal working hours when support staff are available to assist.

13. *The correct answer is C.* Only the clinician should set up local syringes, to reduce the incidence of inoculation injuries. The X-ray machine should never be switched on until its use is imminent, as a faulty machine could be emitting X-rays into the environment all day otherwise and exposing staff to dangerously high levels of emissions. The day list should be checked at the start of the day to ensure all instruments, equipment and laboratory items are present, and the DUWLs must be run through before being used on the first patient.

4a Practice Management and Leadership

Multiple choice questions

1. A person who exhibits good leadership skills tends to be able to influence others positively, by acting as a good role model and setting good examples of how to behave and conduct oneself both professionally and otherwise. Which one of the following options is a leadership skill that is likely to encourage team members to wish to perform well and advance themselves?
   A Ability to act professionally
   B Ability to communicate at several levels
   C Ability to inspire others
   D Ability to take control
   E Ability to take due criticism

2. The specific roles required to achieve good management and leadership of the dental team are set out as guidance by the General Dental Council in their publication *Standards for the Dental Team*. Which one of the following options is a policy that should be in place to ensure that team members are aware of their responsibilities in relation to maintaining and updating their knowledge of various relevant topics?
   A Continuing Professional Development Policy
   B Equality and Diversity Policy
   C Performance Management Policy
   D Raising Concerns Policy
   E Safeguarding Policy

3. All members of the dental team should receive information from the workplace about its correct functioning when they initially begin their role as a team member. This applies whether they are registrants or not and whether they are employed or self-employed. Which one of the following options is the term used to describe this initiation process?
   A Appraisal
   B Continuing professional development

Questions and Answers for Dental Nurses, Fourth Edition. Carole Hollins.

C Equality and diversity
D Induction
E Performance management

4. Part of the role of the practice manager is to direct and organise the dental team so that the workplace runs efficiently and members carry out their roles and responsibilities correctly. On a regular basis the practice manager should provide team members with the opportunity to discuss any issues and comment on their overall performance as a team member. Which one of the following options is the correct term for this feedback process?
   A Appraisal
   B Audit
   C Development
   D Risk assessment
   E Training

5. A person who exhibits good leadership skills tends to be able to influence others positively, by acting as a good role model and setting good examples of how to behave and conduct oneself both professionally and otherwise. Which one of the following options is a leadership skill that allows a person to discuss dental treatments effectively so that informed consent can be given?
   A Ability to act professionally
   B Ability to communicate at several levels
   C Ability to inspire others
   D Ability to take control
   E Ability to take due criticism

6. The specific roles required to achieve good management and leadership of the dental team are set out as guidance by the General Dental Council in their publication *Standards for the Dental Team*. Which one of the following options is a policy that should be in place to ensure that team members know what to do in the event of a performance issue about one of their colleagues?
   A Continuing Professional Development Policy
   B Equality and Diversity Policy
   C Performance Management Policy
   D Raising Concerns Policy
   E Safeguarding Policy

7. A well-run dental workplace should undertake regular staff meetings to ensure that good communication exists between management personnel and dental team members. Which one of the following options is an area of discussion that should not be discussed in staff meetings?
   A Complaints
   B Disciplinary events
   C Policy updates

D Safeguarding issues
E Significant event analysis

8. Part of the management and leadership role is to introduce new policies and procedures, or update existing ones, as necessary from time to time. These should be brought to staff meetings for discussion with all of the dental team members before becoming operative in the workplace. Which one of the following options is not a reason for new policies and procedures to be discussed in this way?
A Ensure compliance with regulations
B Ensure staff understanding of responsibilities
C Obtain approval from team
D Obtain individual compliance
E Opportunity to ask questions

9. When a new member of staff joins the dental team, the practice manager should compile a personnel folder for the individual that acts as a repository for their personal information and legally required documentation. Which one of the following options is an example of copied documentation held in the personnel folder that will provide proof of identity of the individual?
A Curriculum vitae
B Disclosure and Barring Service certificate
C General Dental Council registration certificate
D Indemnity insurance
E Passport

10. A person who exhibits good leadership skills tends to be able to influence others positively, by acting as a good role model and setting good examples of how to behave and conduct oneself both professionally and otherwise. Which one of the following options is a leadership skill that enables a person to learn positively from mistakes, for the benefit of others in the future?
A Ability to act professionally
B Ability to communicate at several levels
C Ability to inspire others
D Ability to take control
E Ability to take due criticism

11. The specific roles required to achieve good management and leadership of the dental team are set out as guidance by the General Dental Council in their publication *Standards for the Dental Team*. Which one of the following options is a policy that should be in place to ensure that team members have a course of action to follow if they have concerns about the welfare of a young patient?
A Continuing Professional Development Policy
B Equality and Diversity Policy
C Performance Management Policy

D Raising Concerns Policy
E Safeguarding Policy

12. A person who exhibits good leadership skills tends to be able to influence others positively, by acting as a good role model and setting good examples of how to behave and conduct oneself both professionally and otherwise. Which one of the following options is a leadership skill that allows a person to successfully organise the dental team during a medical emergency?
    A Ability to act professionally
    B Ability to communicate at several levels
    C Ability to inspire others
    D Ability to take control
    E Ability to take due criticism

13. When a new member of staff joins the dental team, the practice manager should compile a personnel folder for the individual that acts as a repository for their personal information and legally required documentation. Which one of the following options is copied documentation that provides relevant information in the event of a patient complaint against the individual?
    A Curriculum vitae
    B Disclosure and Barring Service certificate
    C General Dental Council registration certificate
    D Indemnity insurance
    E Passport

Extended matching questions

For each of the following teamwork, management and leadership questions, select the single most appropriate answer from the option list. Each option might be used once, more than once or not at all.

a) Attainable
b) Delegation
c) Evaluation
d) Leadership
e) Management
f) Opportunities and threats
g) Professionalism
h) Reflection
i) Specific
j) Strengths and weaknesses
k) Teamwork
l) Verifiable

1. Good management and leadership within the dental workplace should result in efficient delegation of duties amongst staff. This then enables work time to be

used much more effectively throughout the day, as several patients can receive differing levels of care at the same time, and more patients can be attended to within the day. Which one of the options listed is the term used to describe this method of efficient working?

2. An effectively managed dental workplace gives all staff the opportunity to discuss issues that may affect their performance in the workplace, usually as an annual event during a staff appraisal. Which one of the options listed is the term used to describe the external factors affecting a staff member that may be identified during an appraisal?

3. Good teamwork within the dental workplace involves everyone working safely and in harmony so that the end result of their actions is greater and more productive than if they each worked alone. Which one of the options listed is the term used to describe the system where several staff are enabled to provide specific care to a patient in line with their scope of practice, thus achieving good teamwork?

4. A person exhibiting good leadership skills is one who has the ability to always behave in the correct way both while working and in private. They therefore set a good example for others to follow and should be seen as inspirational in encouraging others to improve themselves and achieve their goals. Which one of the options listed is the term used to describe these abilities in a good leader?

5. Sometimes a staff member can display an instinctive ability to influence others in the workplace to want to perform well and emulate the behaviour and conduct of that staff member. Which one of the options listed is the term used to describe this beneficial skill?

6. One of the requirements of a well-led dental workplace is to ensure that all staff have access to opportunities to update their knowledge by attending continuing professional development events. Many organisations run such events, both face to face and online, and staff need to ensure that they are linked to the GDC development outcomes and that an outside body quality assures it. Which one of the options listed is the type of continuing professional development provided when these conditions are met?

7. An effectively managed dental workplace gives all staff the opportunity to discuss issues that may affect their performance in the workplace, usually as an annual event during a staff appraisal. Which one of the options listed is the term used to describe the personal issues affecting a staff member that may be identified during an appraisal?

8. Within the dental workplace it is usual to have a person who acts to direct and organise the team so that the workplace runs efficiently and each member carries out their roles and responsibilities correctly. Which one of the options listed is the term used to describe this person's actions?

Answers

Multiple choice questions

1. *The correct answer is C.* Good leadership is to act as the role model for others to desire to follow and emulate, especially by setting good examples of how to behave and conduct oneself, both professionally and otherwise. It is often an innate, instinctive ability that influences others to want to perform well, push themselves and achieve their goals in life.

2. *The correct answer is A.* The aim of continuing professional development is to achieve lifelong learning. Dentistry is the same as any other profession – new techniques and materials are constantly being developed, some techniques and materials become obsolete or require upgrading to improve patient safety or treatment success and so on. All team members have a duty of care to their patients and colleagues to ensure they stay abreast of all of these developments and updates in a continuous cycle, throughout their career.

3. *The correct answer is D.* A lay person may think that all dental workplaces run in exactly the same way, but nothing could be further from the truth. Every workplace will have carried out its own set of risk assessments and developed its policies from their findings. These will vary between workplaces – a two-surgery, family run practice will operate quite differently from a 10-surgery practice run by a Corporate, for example. Team members must be trained to work correctly in each environment as soon as they arrive – that is the purpose of the induction process.

4. *The correct answer is A.* Appraisals should be carried out annually for every staff member, using standardised appraisal templates that both the staff member and the practice manager can complete beforehand. This gives the employer the opportunity to provide an honest performance review of the staff member, while the staff member has the opportunity to discuss any issues or learning needs in an organised fashion.

5. *The correct answer is B.* Most dental teams provide oral healthcare to a range of age groups and to patients from a variety of backgrounds. The ability to communicate effectively with all patients comes easier to some dental staff than others – some have an inherent ability to communicate well, while others need to learn the skill. Training courses are widely available and should be undertaken where necessary, as good communication is the key to good teamwork and to informed, happy patients.

6. *The correct answer is D.* Throughout the working life of a dental team member, a certain standard of behaviour and competence is expected of them by both the public and the regulators – this is professionalism. When the standards of one team member fall below those expected and patient safety may be at risk, all other team members have a duty to raise concerns about that colleague. The correct actions to take and who to contact about the issue should be written in the Raising Concerns Policy of the workplace.

7. *The correct answer is B.* Disciplinary events are personal and will usually involve one staff member and the employer or manager only. They should not be discussed with other staff members, whether in a meeting or not, unless a safety issue arises. All other options are areas of discussion that should always be discussed in staff meetings.

8. *The correct answer is C.* Introducing a new policy or updating an existing one is purely a management and leadership responsibility, as part of the roles of the manager and team leader is to stay abreast of all the latest advice, guidance, regulations and legislation involved with running the dental workplace. New policies or updated policies are a necessity, not an option, so staff approval of them is not required.

9. *The correct answer is E.* Documentation held for proof of identity purposes must show a current (no older than 10 years) photograph of the named person. Of the options listed, only a passport provides this.

10. *The correct answer is E.* Generally, people do not like to be criticised, but sometimes that criticism is valid, and important points can be learned from it so that people change themselves or how they work for the better. This type of criticism is called constructive as it should produce a positive result by being given and received. Undue criticism is that given unjustly or unfairly, where a person is blamed for something that they are not responsible for.

11. *The correct answer is E.* Safeguarding is the term used to describe the actions required to protect those who cannot protect themselves – children and vulnerable adults. They need protecting from abuse or neglect by another person, for their own safety and welfare. All members of the dental team should be aware of the correct actions to take and the correct organisations to contact in the event of a safeguarding issue – the information should be held in the Safeguarding Policy.

12. *The correct answer is D.* Of all the instants when a person needs the ability to take control and lead others successfully, the medical emergency situation is probably the most important as someone's life may depend upon it. Many dentists are not good team leaders and the role may fall to another member of staff, such as the practice manager or a dental therapist. Whoever, they must stay calm, think logically and organise the rest of the team effectively during the emergency.

13. *The correct answer is D.* All staff members who require registration with the General Dental Council must also have current indemnity insurance too, so that in the event of a patient complaint the matter can be thoroughly investigated without the patient having to pay legal fees to do so. Indemnity insurance requires renewing annually.

Extended matching questions

1. *The correct answer is k).* Teamwork involves staff working together successfully to provide care for their patients. All should work in accordance with the policies of the workplace, respect each member of the team and their role in the workplace and treat each other fairly.

2. *The correct answer is f).* Opportunities are beneficial external factors that may be used to improve the performance of the staff member, such as a supportive employer who is keen to assist staff in achieving further qualifications. Threats are harmful external factors, or obstacles in the way of the staff member that prevent one from improving performance. Examples include poor leadership within the workplace so there is no incentive to improve, or a lack of training opportunities so staff members feel stifled in their role.

3. *The correct answer is b).* A dentist can carry out all necessary treatments for a patient while all other registrants cannot. Good teamwork involves certain of those treatments being delegated to other registrants within their scope of practice, while the dentist proceeds to provide treatments exclusive to their registrant group. For example, the dentist carries out a crown preparation procedure while the therapist restores a deciduous tooth, the hygienist completes a scale and polish and the dental nurse takes impressions for a set of study models. This is the art of good delegation.

4. *The correct answer is g).* All registrants are considered as 'professionals' both by the regulators and by the public, but this is not an automatic right upon qualification and registration. Professionalism involves always doing the right thing and being seen to do so, so that colleagues, the public and the regulators have confidence and trust in that person at all times.

5. *The correct answer is d).* People who are good leaders are able to make others feel good about themselves and feel that they want to perform well and do their best too. They provide inspiration for others to have aims and encourage them to want to achieve their goals.

6. *The correct answer is l).* Only verifiable continuing professional development events count towards the compulsory hours requirements set by the GDC for each registrant group when making an annual CPD declaration. Staff are still encouraged to complete non-verifiable activities such as reading journals and textbooks but must not include the time spent doing these into their CPD activity log.

7. *The correct answer is j).* The strengths of the staff member are those good points personal to them that improve their performance in the workplace, such as reliability or having ambition to achieve a goal. The weaknesses of the staff member are those bad points personal to them that affect their performance detrimentally, such as poor time keeping or lack of ambition.

8. *The correct answer is e).* The person acting as manager may not necessarily be involved in clinical decision making but focuses more on the day-to-day administrative and functional areas of the workplace. The role is often held by a senior member of staff other than a dentist, such as a practice manager.

5 Health and Safety

Multiple choice questions

1. There are several hazardous occupational chemicals used in dentistry, obvious examples being mercury (and amalgam), acid etchant and various cleaning and infection control chemicals including bleach. Which one of the following options is a hazard of spilling acid etchant onto the facial skin of a patient?
   A Corrosive
   B Flammable
   C Irritant
   D Oxidising
   E Toxic

2. All student dental nurses begin their careers working in a supervised environment, either in general practice or in specialist clinics or hospitals. A specific risk assessment will have been carried out to ensure their safety within that environment while carrying out potentially hazardous work activities. Which one of the following options is the most likely activity that could result in the student dental nurse receiving a scald injury?
   A Chairside assisting
   B Instrument decontamination
   C Use of autoclave
   D Use of chemicals
   E Use of X-rays

3. If a fire breaks out in the dental workplace, trained staff may be able to safely extinguish it using suitable firefighting equipment on the premises, so that the risk to all other persons is reduced. Which one of the following options is an example of firefighting equipment that is not suitable for tackling an electrical fire on the premises?
   A Carbon dioxide extinguisher
   B Dry powder extinguisher
   C Foam extinguisher

Questions and Answers for Dental Nurses, Fourth Edition. Carole Hollins.

D Sand
E Water extinguisher

4. Manual handling is the term used to describe any actions that involve the hands-on moving or lifting of items without equipment support. In the dental workplace it usually involves the movement of stock items around the premises, although it may also involve moving patients. Which one of the options listed is a manual handling hazard that can be overcome by splitting the load?
   A Frequency of movement
   B Heavy load
   C High storage shelf
   D Pushing/pulling the load
   E Twisting to carry

5. To ensure a dental workplace is compliant with all of the legal and regulatory requirements involved in its safe running, information must be gathered about the work practices and running of the workplace that are analysed and adjusted as necessary. Once agreed, they become a 'code of conduct' for that workplace. Which one of the options listed is most likely to be the first stage of this process?
   A Agreed protocol
   B Audit
   C Risk assessment
   D Standard operating procedures
   E Written policy

6. The purpose of a risk assessment in the dental workplace is to identify all of the hazards present and reduce or eliminate them so that the workplace is as safe as possible for everyone, while the normal daily work activities are being carried out. Which one of the following options is most likely to be the second stage of the assessment process?
   A Control the risk
   B Evaluate the risk
   C Identify the hazard
   D Identify who may be harmed
   E Record the findings

7. In line with Ionising Radiation regulations 2017 (IRR17) and Ionising Regulations (Medical Exposure) Regulations 2017 (IR(ME)R17), various roles and formal appointments must be made by all dental workplaces using X-ray machines in their premises. Which one of the following options is the title of the person who may carry out a radiation survey for the workplace and ensure new machines are installed correctly?
   A IR(ME)R17 practitioner
   B Operator
   C Radiation protection advisor
   D Radiation protection supervisor
   E Referrer

8. The Control of Substances Hazardous to Health 2002 (COSHH) regulations require all dental workplaces to carry out a COSHH risk assessment of all chemicals and potentially hazardous substances used or held on the premises, to identify those that may cause harm. A hazard classification can then be assigned to the substance using the internationally recognised hazard symbols – currently red-bordered white diamonds with a black pictogram within. Which one of the options listed is the pictogram indicating a substance is toxic or very toxic?
   A Dead tree and fish
   B Exclamation mark
   C Flame
   D Flame surrounding a circle
   E Skull and crossbones

9. A written emergency plan is used to guide all staff in the actions to take in the event of a fire on the premises. It must contain clear written instructions on various points and also must be accessible to all staff at all times. Which one of the following options is written information that is not required in an emergency plan?
   A Assembly point
   B Attendance check procedures
   C Key escape routes
   D Location of smoke alarms
   E Warning system in use

10. The waste produced by a dental workplace is categorised as non-hazardous, hazardous infectious or hazardous chemical waste in line with the Department of Health's HTM 07-01 document *Safe Management of Healthcare Waste* (2013). Which one of the following options is the correct waste receptacle for the storage and disposal of contaminated PPE items?
   A Blue/yellow tub with blue lid
   B Orange sack
   C Yellow sack with black stripe
   D Yellow tub
   E Yellow tub with purple lid

11. The use of computers in the dental workplace is now commonplace, and employers are required to make certain provisions for staff under the Health and Safety (Display Screen Equipment) Regulations to avoid any ill effects while using them. Which one of the options listed is an issue most likely to result in eye strain for the computer user?
   A Anti-glare screen
   B Bright screen
   C Chair too high
   D No footrest
   E Small workspace

12. Under the most recent fire safety regulations, it is the employer's responsibility to take reasonable steps to reduce the risk from fire in their work premises by carrying out a fire risk assessment. The fire precautions required will vary from one workplace to another, but the risk assessment process is always the same. Which one of the options listed is the stage where any necessary changes or updates to the risk assessment are identified and put into action?
    A Control the risk
    B Evaluate the risk
    C Identify the hazard
    D Identify who may be harmed
    E Review the findings

13. If a significant event occurs in the dental workplace, it is classed as a notifiable incident and must be reported to the Health and Safety Executive (HSE) within a set time frame. Which one of the following options is not classed as a significant event and therefore need not be reported to HSE?
    A Amputation of hand
    B Clean needlestick injury
    C Compressor explosion
    D Fractured femur
    E Infection with human immunodeficiency virus

14. The mains water supply to the dental workplace is held in the plumbing system – the hot- and cold-water storage tanks and the pipework running between the two and around the premises. Legionella may grow and proliferate anywhere in this system if the water temperature regularly lies within a certain range. Which one of the following options is the optimal temperature range within which Legionella can proliferate within the plumbing system of the premises?
    A Above 15°C to below 40°C
    B Above 15°C to below 45°C
    C Above 20°C to below 45°C
    D Above 20°C to below 55°C
    E Above 25°C to below 50°C

15. There is always some degree of cell damage caused when a patient undergoes exposure to X-rays, and it is therefore accepted that there is no 'safe' level of exposure. Consequently, strict legislation and guidelines must be complied with by all dental workplaces when X-rays are in use. Which one of the following options is the term used in radiography to determine that the benefits of X-ray exposure outweigh the risks to the patient?
    A Identification
    B Justification
    C Optimisation
    D Quality assurance
    E Referrer

Extended matching questions

Topic: I

For each of the following health and safety questions, select the single most appropriate answer from the option list. Each option might be used once, more than once or not at all.

a) Audit
b) Control the risk
c) Evaluate the risk
d) Identify the hazard
e) Identify who may be harmed
f) Policy
g) Quality assurance
h) Record the findings
i) Risk assessment
j) Standard operating procedures

1. A dental practice has carried out a fire safety risk assessment and identified an issue with their fire extinguisher maintenance programme. In effect, the pressure gauge on the foam extinguishers was not being checked regularly by any staff member, and one extinguisher was found to be unusable in the event of a fire. Consequently, the practice set out a written course of action to be followed by all staff in relation to fire safety management for the premises. Which one of the options listed is the correct term for this written course of action?

2. Every 6 months a member of staff is tasked with the job of randomly choosing 10 patients who have attended the practice for a dental examination and checking the written records that were made at the time of the appointment. The staff member is determining whether notes were made under each of the sub-headings of the dental examination template as necessary, such as whether the medical history was updated, whether a written report was made if any X-rays were taken and that a written treatment plan was made. Which one of the options listed is the correct term for this process of checking procedures and analysing the results achieved?

3. The practice has decided to begin using a different surface disinfectant from the current one, as it is more readily available from suppliers. While checking the COSHH information supplied with the new product, it is noted that the solution has a warning of giving off strong vapours that may cause airway irritation if inhaled. Which one of the options listed is the stage of a risk assessment that will determine if the product is safe to be used in the premises and if it only poses a risk if misused?

Topic: II

For each of the following health and safety questions, select the single most appropriate answer from the option list. Each option might be used once, more than once or not at all.

a) Control of Substances Hazardous to Health 2002
b) Hazardous Waste Regulations 2005
c) Health and Safety (First Aid) Regulations 1981
d) Ionising Radiation (Medical Exposures) Regulations 2017
e) Ionising Radiation Regulations 2017
f) Management of Health and Safety at Work Regulations 1999
g) Pressure Systems Safety Regulations 2000
h) Regulatory Reform (Fire Safety) Order 2005
i) Reporting of Injuries, Diseases and Dangerous Occurrences Regulations 2013

1. All dental workplaces have numerous items of electrical equipment and appliances on the premises, along with many hazardous chemicals that may cause harm if used incorrectly. Which one of the options listed is legislation that requires the workplace to have an emergency plan in place, in the event of a dangerous occurrence such as an explosion or a leak of hazardous fumes?

2. The use of X-rays in the dental workplace provides a valuable diagnostic tool for the dental team and assists in the successful treatment of dental disease in patients. However, it is accepted that there is no safe level of exposure to X-rays, and their use is therefore subject to specific legislation for both staff and patients. Which one of the options listed is the set of regulations that must be followed to ensure the safety and protection of patients while undergoing radiation procedures?

3. During a quiet period at the practice, one of the staff is tasked with emptying the automatic X-ray processing machine and carrying out a thorough cleaning of the tanks and rollers. During the cleaning process, it is discovered that the developer drum is already full so the chemical is disposed of into the sink instead, followed by a thorough swilling with tap water. Which one of the options listed is the legislation that has been breached by the staff member in this scenario?

Answers

Multiple choice questions

1. *The correct answer is A.* Acid etchant (as the name suggests) is an acidic product that is therefore capable of chemically burning soft tissues and skin if spilled. It should only be placed on the tooth itself during use and carefully irrigated off and aspirated away without any soft tissue contact.

2. *The correct answer is C.* When the door of an autoclave is opened immediately after a cycle has been completed, steam billows out of the chamber and can scald anyone standing in front of the autoclave. A scald is a burn caused by hot liquid or steam.

3. *The correct answer is E.* Water applied to a source of electricity (any electrical item in the workplace) is likely to cause the electrocution of the person applying the water to the fire. Electricity cannot travel through air, but it can through water and the use of water on an electrical item is similar to putting your fingers into a live electrical socket. Both carbon dioxide and dry foam extinguishers can be used safely on electrical fires.

4. *The correct answer is B.* Often, dental supplies are delivered to the workplace contained in one large box for ease of transport by the courier. However, they are often heavy when packaged in this way and are likely to cause muscle strain or injury if staff attempt to move large, heavy boxes around the workplace. Instead, the load should be opened at the point of delivery and split into several smaller loads that are easier and safer to carry.

5. *The correct answer is C.* Initially, a risk assessment is carried out to identify what hazards or potential hazards exist in the workplace itself and while carrying out the day-to-day procedures within the workplace. Once identified, the hazards can be reduced or removed as necessary so that a working policy can be produced.

6. *The correct answer is D.* Initially the hazard must be identified, and then those who may be harmed by that hazard should be identified. For example, the use of a particular chemical to disinfect laboratory work has been identified as a hazard because it gives off fumes, but it will only be a hazard to those staff specifically involved in its use, not to other staff such as those who are involved in administrative work only.

7. *The correct answer is C.* The radiation protection advisor is a radiation specialist who is formally appointed by the dental workplace to give advice on staff and public safety. Under IR(ME)R17 they advise on the correct installation of new X-ray machines by carrying out acceptance testing of the machines.

8. *The correct answer is E.* The skull and crossbones symbol indicates the chemical will cause death if mishandled (such as mercury).

9. *The correct answer is D.* The positioning of smoke alarms around the workplace should have been advised upon at the initial fire inspection, but their location does not need to be recorded in the emergency plan as it is irrelevant to the safe evacuation of the premises in an emergency. All other options are relevant to the emergency plan being followed correctly and safely.

10. *The correct answer is B.* All clinical bins should be lined with an orange sack provided by the workplace's certificated hazardous waste collection company. All used PPE items should be placed in these receptacles after use (masks, gloves, visors, gowns, etc.) with all other soft clinical waste. When full, the sacks should be tied, removed to a secure area and labelled with the workplace address ready for collection and disposal by the waste company.

11. *The correct answer is B.* All computers in use at the dental workplace should have functioning brightness and contrast controls so that the screen can be adjusted to suit the user. A bright screen makes the eye muscles work harder to keep the pupil size small so that excess light does not enter the eyes – the muscles will become overtired and cause eye strain.

12. *The correct answer is E.* All risk assessments should be reviewed on a regular basis, say once every 2 years unless an incident has occurred that prompts an earlier review. The review should reconsider the original risk assessment findings and action plan and determine if they are still applicable to the workplace or if any changes or updates are required. Changes or updates may be required if relevant legislation has altered, or if an incident has occurred that showed the systems in place to reduce the risk have failed.

13. *The correct answer is B.* A clean needlestick injury is one where an unused (sterile) item has pierced the skin of the victim, causing injury but no possibility of infection transmission. The event requires analysis to determine how it happened and to prevent a recurrence by changing the necessary protocol, but it is not classed as a significant event requiring formal reporting and investigation.

14. *The correct answer is C.* Cold water below 20°C and hot water above 45°C are outside the temperature range for Legionella to survive. Hence, monthly checks of the workplace's cold and hot water tap temperatures should be carried out and recorded to ensure that these parameters are not breached. If they are, the workplace must follow their Legionella management policy to deal with the issue.

15. *The correct answer is B.* Under IR(ME)R 2017, every exposure is expected to provide new information to assist with diagnosis, treatment or prognosis, otherwise there is no sound reason to be carrying out the exposure. This is termed the 'justification' for the exposure and should be recorded in the patient's notes. There is no such thing as 'routine X-rays' in a modern dental workplace.

Extended matching questions

Topic: I

1. *The correct answer is f).* A policy document should be written after a risk assessment has been carried out in the workplace. It should state the courses of action that have been adopted by the workplace in relation to various activities (in this scenario a fire safety management policy) and must be read, agreed upon, signed by all staff to accept its content and then followed at all times by all staff.
2. *The correct answer is a).* Audits should be carried out in various areas of dentistry on a regular basis, as it should be a cyclical process of continual assessment and improvement. The aim is to assess the quality and effectiveness of certain areas of the service delivered to patients, determine if the workplace policies are followed correctly and good quality is assured or determine how to improve the systems in place to provide a better service in future. The same service should then be re-examined at a later date to ensure the quality is being maintained or further improved – hence the term 'audit cycle'.
3. *The correct answer is c).* Initially the risk must be identified, and then those at risk can be identified. So, in this scenario the risk is a health and safety issue, and it may affect anyone using the product. The next stage of the risk assessment is to evaluate the product and determine if there is a risk every time it is used, or only if it is mishandled (for example, spilled), or only if certain precautions required during its use are not followed (for example, not wearing the correct PPE during use).

Topic: II

1. *The correct answer is h).* This legislation requires the 'responsible person' (employer or owner of the premises) to take reasonable steps to reduce the risk from fire within the premises and to ensure that anyone in the premises can escape safely if there is a fire or other significant event that may lead to a fire (gas leak, electrical fault, explosion, etc.). This is achieved by carrying out an initial risk assessment and then formulating a written emergency plan for evacuating the premises and all persons within, including arrangements for disabled, child and elderly patients. Reporting of Injuries, Diseases and Dangerous Occurrences Regulations (RIDDOR) is concerned with the correct reporting of such incidents to the Health and Safety Executive.
2. *The correct answer is d).* These regulations were updated in 2017 and are specifically concerned with the safety of patients in the dental workplace and with the protection of patients, carers and comforters during exposure to ionising radiation. Ionising Radiation Regulations 2017 (IRR17) are concerned with the safety and protection of staff in the dental workplace where ionising radiation is used.

3. *The correct answer is b).* All dental workplaces have a statutory duty of care to ensure they avoid cross-infection of people and cross-contamination of the environment by managing and disposing of healthcare waste in accordance with these regulations. Processing chemicals are classed as hazardous chemical waste and must be stored on the premises in suitable drums before collection by a certificated hazardous waste collection company. They are toxic to wildlife and vegetation and must never be disposed of via the drains.

6 Medical Emergencies and First Aid

Multiple choice questions

1. There are several diagnosed medical conditions that a patient may have that should alert the dental team to the potential increased risk of that patient suffering a medical emergency while undergoing dental treatment. Which one of the following risk factors may result in an anxious patient suffering a cardiac arrest?
   A Asthma
   B Dementia
   C Diabetes
   D Hepatitis
   E Hypertension

2. When patients begin to show signs of becoming unwell, they must be quickly and methodically assessed by the dental team to determine the correct actions to be taken. Which one of the following is the correct abbreviated approach for this assessment?
   A ABCDE
   B AED
   C BLS
   D CPR
   E DRSABC

3. An automated external defibrillator (AED) is a device used to 'shock', or defibrillate, a casualty's malfunctioning heart muscle during a medical emergency. Which one of the following statements is incorrect in relation to the accurate use of the AED during an emergency?
   A Continue CPR while pads are applied
   B Press the 'shock' button when prompted
   C Remove oxygen supply before shocking
   D Remove pads if 'shock' not prompted
   E Stop CPR after pads are applied

Questions and Answers for Dental Nurses, Fourth Edition. Carole Hollins.

4. When assessing the responsiveness (or level of disability) of a casualty, the rescuer should quickly follow the abbreviated ACVPU system. Which one of the following indicates that the casualty is unable to tell rescuers where they are or how they arrived there?
   A Alert
   B Confused
   C Painful
   D Unresponsive
   E Verbal

5. When a casualty is found collapsed, the rescuer must quickly assess the situation and determine what they can safely do to assist the casualty, in line with the DRSABC approach. Which one of the following findings should alert the rescuer to prepare to administer basic life support (BLS) to the casualty?
   A Abnormal breathing
   B Arterial bleeding
   C Fractured leg
   D Rapid pulse
   E Tonic-clonic seizure

6. An automated external defibrillator (AED) is a device used to 'shock', or defibrillate, a casualty's malfunctioning heart muscle during a medical emergency. Which one of the following options is unlikely to affect the correct functioning of the AED while in use?
   A Damp skin
   B Hairy chest
   C No mains electric supply
   D Pads applied to clothing
   E Right side pad placed at heart apex

7. On finding a collapsed casualty, the rescuer should assess the situation by following the DRSABC approach to determine if the casualty is fully unconscious and whether they are breathing or not. Which one of the following options is a correct statement when the casualty is a collapsed baby or young child?
   A Do not use the AED
   B Give 30 compressions then 5 rescue breaths
   C Give 5 back slaps
   D Give 5 rescue breaths before starting compressions
   E Use a 15:2 algorithm

8. When an incident occurs in the dental workplace that requires the administration of first aid, it is important for trained staff members to carry out that first aid in a timely and ordered manner. Which one of the following listed actions should be the first to take after a patient slips off the stairs and suffers a compound fracture of the leg?

A Apply a splint
B Apply a tourniquet
C Cover the exposed bone
D Straighten the leg
E Wash the wound

9. Sometimes casualties collapse but maintain their own airway and circulation, and the rescuer then needs to carefully move them into the recovery position until specialist help arrives. Which one of the following options listed should be the rescuer's last action to take when putting the casualty into the recovery position?
A Bend the nearest arm up
B Bend the upper leg
C Put furthest hand against the face
D Roll the casualty towards them
E Tilt the head back

10. The ability to recognise the signs and symptoms of the various causes of collapse is an essential skill for all members of the dental team, including dental nurses. Of the potential causes of collapse in the dental surgery, which one of the following is most likely to respond to the administration of intramuscular adrenaline by a trained member of the dental team?
A Anaphylaxis
B Angina attack
C Choking episode
D Diabetic coma
E Myocardial infarction

11. When the dental team are faced with an unwell or collapsed casualty, the successful treatment or resuscitation of that casualty will depend on the recognition of the signs and symptoms of the event and the correct differential diagnosis of the actual cause of the collapse. When the rescuer notices the casualty has slurred speech, which one of the following pairs of medical emergencies should be considered as possible causes for the emergency?
A Angina attack and epileptic fit
B Asthma attack and diabetic coma
C Hypoglycaemia and stroke
D Myocardial infarction and anaphylaxis
E Stroke and adrenal crisis

12. In line with Health and Safety at Work requirements, the dental workplace must have adequate provision to administer first aid when necessary. Which one of the following first aid events is most likely to occur when a staff member touches a faulty curing light plug with wet hands?
A Burn
B Electrocution

C Fracture
D Poisoning
E Scald

13. When an incident occurs in the dental workplace that requires the administration of first aid, it is important for trained staff members to carry out that first aid in a timely and ordered manner. Which one of the following listed actions should be the first to take when a staff member accidently cuts a hand open when about to use a sharp item?
A Apply a tourniquet
B Apply antiseptic soap
C Apply direct pressure
D Check COSHH folder for advice
E Wash in warm water

14. When a patient begins to feel unwell, the dental team should quickly assess the various signs and symptoms that the patient is experiencing to determine the likely cause of the problem, so that suitable treatment can be given. Which one of the following combinations of signs and symptoms is most likely to indicate the onset of an asthma attack?
A Cyanosis, difficulty breathing
B Hypotension, nausea
C Irregular pulse, chest pain
D Pale, feeling dizzy
E Stridor, difficulty breathing

15. When assessing a collapsed casualty using the DRSABC approach, the rescuer will assess the rate and quality of any breath sounds to help determine the cause of the collapse. Which one of the following would indicate the presence of fluid in the airways, such as vomit or excess mucus secretions?
A Gasping
B Rattling
C Snoring
D Stridor
E Wheezing

Extended matching questions

Topic: I

For each of the following medical emergency –signs and symptoms questions, select the single most appropriate answer from the option list. Each option might be used once, more than once or not at all.

a) Chest pain and facial congestion
b) Coughing and cyanotic

c) Cyanotic and unable to speak
d) Disorientated and unable to speak
e) Dizzy and clammy skin
f) Drowsy and irritable
g) Facial swelling and breathless
h) Gasping breathlessness and stridor
i) Grey pallor and not breathing
j) Low blood pressure and fast pulse
k) Severe headache and irritable
l) Slurred speech and facial droop
m) Unresponsive and convulsions
n) Wheezing and cyanotic

1. A patient attends the practice for a routine dental examination but becomes unwell during the procedure. He is known to suffer from type II diabetes, and the dental team suspect he is hypoglycaemic. Which one of the options listed is the most likely combination of signs and/or symptoms to indicate this medical emergency?

2. A nervous patient is overdue for a dental appointment and on checking, the receptionist finds him in a distressed state within the entrance foyer of the practice. She suspects the patient is having an angina attack and raises the alarm with her colleagues. Which one of the options listed is the most likely combination of signs and/or symptoms to indicate this medical emergency?

3. While walking to the practice one morning, the hygienist comes across a collapsed casualty in the street. She calls for paramedics and is able to suggest to the operator that the casualty is having an epileptic seizure. Which one of the options listed is the most likely combination of signs and/or symptoms to indicate this medical emergency?

4. A mother and her three young children have attended for their routine dental examinations and go into the surgery one at a time to see the dentist. While the mother is being examined, the youngest child is given a sweet by his sister and suddenly becomes distressed. The receptionist believes he is choking on the sweet and proceeds to assist him. Which one of the options listed is the most likely combination of signs and/or symptoms to indicate this medical emergency?

Topic: II

For each of the following first aid questions, select the single most appropriate answer from the option list. Each option might be used once, more than once, or not at all.

a) Administer back slaps
b) Apply a splint
c) Apply a tourniquet

d) Apply direct pressure
e) Avoid movement
f) Cover the wound
g) Induce vomiting
h) Open the windows
i) Place under cold water
j) Raise the limb
k) Remove jewellery
l) Remove the object
m) Squeeze the wound
n) Straighten the limb
o) Switch off the electric
p) Wash the wound

1. After replacing the blown fuse in a portable appliance, the dentist is returning the screwdriver to the practice toolbox when he trips over and falls with the screwdriver piercing his wrist. The wound immediately begins pumping blood out and his colleagues rush to assist him, carrying out initial first aid steps to stop the arterial bleeding but failing to do so. Which one of the options listed is the most likely first aid action that they should finally take in this scenario?

2. During a restorative procedure a ball of lining material falls to the back of the patient's mouth and lodges in his oropharynx. He quickly sits upright and begins coughing uncontrollably. Which one of the options listed is the most likely first aid action to be taken by the dental team?

3. On leaving the dental practice after his appointment, an elderly patient misses his step onto the pavement and falls over, causing an open fracture to his left forearm as he tries to stop his fall. The dental team rush outside to assist him and see the end of the bone piercing his skin. Which one of the options listed is the most likely first aid action to be taken by the team?

4. During a busy session at the dental practice, one of the surgeries is about to run out of processed instruments so the dental nurse is awaiting the end of the autoclave cycle to retrieve more instruments for that surgery. As soon as the cycle is ended she opens the autoclave door and her hand is enveloped in billowing steam from the appliance. Which one of the options listed is the most likely first aid action to be taken?

Answers

Multiple choice questions

1. *The correct answer is E.* Hypertension is a condition of having a persistently raised blood pressure at rest and results in the heart continually having to work harder to pump blood around the body. Over time this tires out the cardiac muscle tissue, and the heart becomes less effective as a pumping organ and more likely to stop (arrest) when overexerted or during times of increased anxiety.

2. *The correct answer is A.* Airway, Breathing, Circulation, Disability and Exposure are the methodical steps to be checked and observed while assessing the unwell, but still conscious, casualty – and in their order of importance. So the airway should be checked for blockages and made patent before assessing the quality of their breathing, which in turn should be determined before assessing their circulation by monitoring the speed and quality of their pulse, and so on. The DRSABC approach is that to be followed when a patient collapses or is found collapsed.

3. *The correct answer is D.* The AED analyses the heart rhythm once the pads are applied and will not prompt the rescuer to 'shock' unless the heart is fibrillating. Fibrillation is a shockable rhythm, but other heart rhythms such as asystole are not – in these circumstances CPR must continue with the AED still attached, as the CPR efforts may actually stimulate the heart from no activity (asystole) into fibrillation. Once fibrillating, the AED can then 'shock' the heart and hopefully convert the electrical activity into an effective sinus rhythm.

4. *The correct answer is B.* The casualty has a reduced level of consciousness and is still able to talk to rescuers but is making little sense. This may be due to an obvious head injury, or one of several medical emergency situations such as a stroke, or any event causing hypoxia or hypotension. It may also be due to alcohol or drug ingestion.

5. *The correct answer is A.* Any abnormal breathing indicates that the casualty is receiving gradually diminishing amounts of oxygen to the brain, due to a blocked airway, a chest injury, a failing heart, etc. Some amount of permanent brain damage will occur if oxygenated blood is not pumped to it within 3–4 minutes, so BLS must begin as soon as possible – starting with chest compressions, then rescue breathing at the current 30:2 algorithm.

6. *The correct answer is C.* All AED devices operate using an internal electrical battery so that they can be used anywhere, indoors or outside, rather than having to be connected to the mains electricity supply via a plug. One of the many daily checks carried out in the dental practice should be to check that the 'battery OK' flashing light is working on the AED, so that it can be safely and effectively used during a medical emergency. A written record should be kept of this check as part of the practice's compliance and due diligence records.

7. *The correct answer is D.* The usual cause of collapse in a young casualty is airway obstruction rather than cardiac arrest, as in an adult. Consequently, a young casualty is likely to have been oxygen-starved for some time before collapsing, so giving 5 rescue breaths into the opened airway before starting compressions will provide much-needed oxygen to the vital organs. Basic life support should then proceed in the usual 30:2 algorithm while the AED is applied and help summoned.

8. *The correct answer is C.* The first aid principle is to prevent further tissue damage by restricting any movement of the casualty and with a compound fracture to also prevent infection of the exposed bone by covering it with a clean dressing. The wound should not be handled otherwise, to minimise the risk of infection, and if bleeding occurs direct pressure should be applied rather than a tourniquet.

9. *The correct answer is E.* The recovery position achieved must be stabilised by the necessary arm, hand and leg movements before the head is finally tilted back to maintain an open airway.

10. *The correct answer is A.* This is a sudden and severe reaction of the casualty's immune system to an allergen, such as penicillin or latex, where they experience swelling of the head and neck tissues and a sudden fall in blood pressure, causing collapse. The swift administration of one or more doses of intramuscular adrenaline may prevent the casualty suffering a cardiac arrest, but they will still require transfer to hospital by paramedics to undergo further treatment and investigations.

11. *The correct answer is C.* A patient suffering from hypoglycaemia often appears confused and drunk with slurred speech, as their blood sugar levels drop too low. One of the classic signs to identify with a patient suspected of having a stroke is that they have altered speech (Face, Arms, Speech, Time to call 999).

12. *The correct answer is B.* Any device connected to the mains electric supply has electrical current running through it when in use. If the plug is faulty (exposed wires, cracked plug casing, etc.), the electric supply is no longer safely enclosed within the plug during use but can discharge into the surrounding environment. Human skin has no resistance to electricity and if wet or damp, electricity can pass through with even greater ease, causing an electric shock or electrocution.

13. *The correct answer is C.* Whether the bleeding is arterial, venous or capillary, the first action to take is to apply direct pressure to the site, ideally with the arm raised above heart level to assist in stemming the blood flow. The wound should not be disturbed by washing, and a tourniquet should only ever be applied as a last resort when a large artery has been severed.

14. *The correct answer is A.* The casualty's airways become narrowed on exposure to inhaled particles, so that exhalation is forced and difficult. The reduced oxygen intake and poor perfusion of the blood with oxygen causes cyanosis that is noticeable in the lips and face.

15. *The correct answer is B.* The 'wet' breathing sounds, or rattle, of a semi-conscious or unconscious casualty are due to a build-up of fluids in the airway that cannot be expelled as normal by coughing. The fluids remain in the airway and cause the rattling, gurgling sound as air is drawn through the partial obstruction.

Extended matching questions

Topic: I

1. *The correct answer is f).* These signs often occur in known diabetics when the blood sugar levels fall, either due to incorrect insulin or carbohydrate intake. The casualty may become combative or appear as if drunk. Oral glucose should be administered while the person is still conscious.

2. *The correct answer is a).* The facial congestion seen during an angina attack is quite the opposite of the pallor and greyness seen when a casualty suffers a myocardial infarction, but both will have some degree of chest pain. The pain may extend into the arm, shoulder or jaw or may be mistaken for indigestion.

3. *The correct answer is m).* During an epileptic seizure the casualty is unconscious and therefore unresponsive and will exhibit tonic-clonic episodes where the person initially becomes rigid and then convulses uncontrollably. The seizure may last less than a minute or become more prolonged or repetitive.

4. *The correct answer is b).* Coughing when a foreign object becomes lodged in the airway is an uncontrollable protective mechanism of the respiratory system, as the body tries to eject the blockage by forcing bursts of air from the lungs outwards. The blockage also prevents oxygen entering the lungs to pass into the blood and circulate around the body, so the blood remains deoxygenated and shows in the lips and nails as cyanosis.

Topic: II

1. *The correct answer is c).* The first aid principle with severe bleeding is to restrict the blood flow to the wound and encourage clotting to reduce blood loss. In this scenario the initial first aid of raising the arm above heart level and applying direct pressure to the wound for around 15 minutes has failed. The final action then is to apply a tourniquet for up to 15 minutes to restrict blood loss from the damaged artery.

2. *The correct answer is a).* Encourage the casualty to lean forwards and then administer up to 5 back slaps, hitting the casualty sharply between the shoulder blades with the flat of the hand. If this fails to dislodge the obstruction then abdominal thrusts must be given.

3. *The correct answer is f).* Open fractures are prone to infection as the bone is exposed to air and possibly dirt from the surroundings. Serious bone infections are likely to complicate the healing of the injured part and may even result in amputation if healing fails. The wound should be covered as soon as possible with a clean (preferably sterile) dressing, such as those stored in the first aid kit.

4. *The correct answer is i).* The dental nurse has suffered a scald to her hand – a wet burn caused by skin contact with the steam from the autoclave. The first aid principles are to reduce blistering and loss of blood serum and prevent infection. The injured part should be immersed into cold water for up to 10 minutes to reduce blistering, and medical attention should be sought for all but a minor scald.

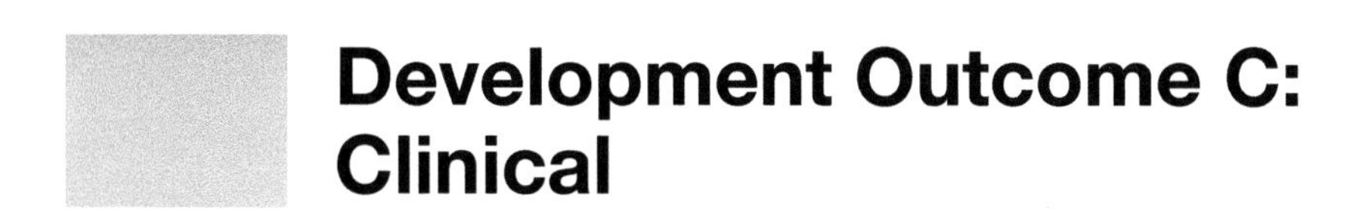

Development Outcome C: Clinical

7 Infection Prevention and Control

Multiple choice questions

1. The oral cavity is teeming with micro-organisms, even in healthy patients, so the need for infection prevention and control in dentistry is of great importance. The basic principle of infection control is to assume that any patient may be infected with any micro-organism at any time and could pose a risk to all dental staff and other patients. Which one of the following is the term used that enshrines this principle of infection control?
   A Direct cross-infection
   B Health and Social Care Act 2008
   C Indirect cross-infection
   D Standard operating procedures
   E Standard precautions

2. The terms 'cleaning' and 'cleanliness' in a clinical context are quite different from those used in general and by lay persons. Which one of the following terms indicates to the dental team the process of killing all micro-organisms and spores?
   A Asepsis
   B Decontamination
   C Disinfection
   D Social cleaning
   E Sterilisation

3. An important aspect of infection prevention and control in the dental workplace is that of re-processing instruments so that they may be safely handled by staff and reused on another patient. It involves several stages that must be carried out in the correct order to achieve the required aim. Which one of the following options should be the first of these stages to be carried out?
   A Cleaning
   B Disinfection
   C Inspection

Questions and Answers for Dental Nurses, Fourth Edition. Carole Hollins.

D Sterilisation
E Storage

4. Effective hand washing is the most important method of preventing cross-infection in any environment but particularly in a clinical setting. The correct method of hand washing is that stipulated by the Health and Safety Council and should be followed whether mild antibacterial liquid soap or alcohol-based hand gel is used. Which one of the following actions is required when using either mild antibacterial liquid soap or alcohol-based hand gel?
   A Apply cleaning product to hands
   B Dry with disposable towels
   C Rinse hands with water
   D Use foot- or elbow-operated sink taps
   E Wet both hands with water

5. Personal protective equipment (PPE) is that worn to prevent contamination of the skin, mucous membranes, airways and clothing of the dental staff by the patient before, during and after dental treatment. Which one of the following items of PPE should be worn to prevent contamination of the mucous membranes of the eyes during an aerosol procedure?
   A FFP2 mask
   B FFP3 mask
   C Full gown
   D Surgical face mask
   E Visor

6. Various equipment items are available for use in the dental workplace to decontaminate reusable hand instruments safely. To ensure that the equipment items work correctly, they should undergo various validation tests on a regular basis, in line with current HTM 01-05 guidance. Which one of the following options is a validation test for washer-disinfectors to ensure that contaminants are effectively removed from instruments during the cycle?
   A Chemical dosing test
   B Foil ablation test
   C Protein residue test
   D Soil efficacy test
   E Steam penetration test

7. In line with the National Patient Safety Agency guidance, cleaning equipment used throughout the dental workplace should be colour-coded so that items are used in specified areas only. This helps prevent the inadvertent transfer of contamination from areas of potentially high infection to areas of low infection. Which one of the following options is the colour-coding of equipment for use in a potentially low infection area, such as the waiting room?

A Blue
B Green
C Red
D White
E Yellow

8. Cleaning of the dental clinical area is especially important following an aerosol generating procedure (AGP), such as restorative treatment or ultrasonic scaling. There are various disinfectant solutions and combinations available for this purpose. Which one of the following options is a cleaning agent that weakens in strength over time so should be made fresh on a regular basis?
   A Alcohol/detergent combined solution
   B Aldehyde-based solution
   C Bleach-based solution
   D Hypochlorous acid solution
   E Isopropyl alcohol solution

9. Dental unit water lines (DUWLs) are the hoses running from the bracket table to the dental handpieces, scaler tip and triple syringe device. Research has shown that DUWLs can become contaminated by micro-organisms if not maintained and cleaned effectively in the dental workplace. Which one of the following options is the correct frequency with which DUWLs should be cleaned with a biocide chemical to prevent biofilm build-up?
   A Every month
   B Every use
   C Every week
   D Once per day
   E Once per session

10. To avoid the build-up of micro-organisms and biofilm in the plumbing system of the dental workplace, monthly recorded temperature performance checks must be carried out. The cold and hot water supplies must be outside the temperature range within which micro-organisms may actively grow. Which one of the following options indicates a temperature performance check record that falls within the micro-organism active growth range?
   A Calorifier at 60°C
   B Cold water at 10°C
   C Cold water at 15°C
   D Hot water at 45°C
   E Hot water at 55°C

11. Effective decontamination and cleaning of dental hand instruments are duties usually carried out by the dental nurse in most small dental workplaces. The aim of the decontamination process is to remove contaminants from reusable items so that they are safe for further use on other patients. Which one of the

following options is the decontamination equipment designed to disinfect hand instruments thermally?

A B-type autoclave
B N-type autoclave
C Nylon bristle-brush
D Ultrasonic bath
E Washer-disinfector

12. Various equipment items are available for use in the dental workplace to decontaminate reusable hand instruments safely. To ensure that the equipment items work correctly, they should undergo various validation tests on a regular basis, in line with current HTM 01-05 guidance. Which one of the following options is a validation test for ultrasonic baths to ensure that all blood contamination has been removed effectively?

A Chemical dosing test
B Foil ablation test
C Protein residue test
D Soil efficacy test
E Steam penetration test

13. Once hand instruments and dental handpieces have completed the reprocessing cycle, they are available for storage or re-use on another patient. Which one of the following options is not a suitable storage regime for these items?

A Unwrapped in clinical area for 1 week
B Unwrapped in clinical area for same day
C Unwrapped in non-clinical area for 1 week
D Wrapped in clinical area for 1 year
E Wrapped in non-clinical area for 1 year

14. All dental workplaces have a statutory duty of care to ensure that they avoid cross-infection of people and cross-contamination of the environment by managing and disposing of all the healthcare waste they produce appropriately. Which one of the following options is an example of items categorised as hazardous infectious waste?

A Expired liner material
B Lead foil
C Scalpel blade and suture needle (used)
D Study model casts
E X-ray fixer solution

15. The close nature of providing dental treatment to patients exposes all clinical dental staff to a variety of micro-organisms daily, as many are spread by direct or indirect contact with body fluids, including the potentially contaminated spray produced during aerosol generating procedures. Which one of the following

options is a serious bacterial infection that causes lung damage and is spread by droplet contamination and direct contact?

A Covid-19
B Creutzfeldt-Jakob disease
C Hepatitis B
D Influenza
E Tuberculosis

16. Various electrical appliances are available for use when re-processing instruments and handpieces in the dental workplace. A good understanding of their modes of operation assists staff in maintaining them correctly and in identifying when faults have occurred. Which one of the following options is an appliance that operates at 134°C for 3 minutes at 2.25 bar pressure with a vacuum?

A B-type autoclave
B Illuminated magnifier
C N-type autoclave
D Ultrasonic bath
E Washer-disinfector

Extended matching questions

Topic: I

For each of the following Infection Prevention and Control Policy (HTM 01-05) questions, select the single most appropriate answer from the option list. Each option might be used once, more than once or not at all.

a) Blood spillage procedure
b) Decontamination of instruments
c) General cleaning
d) Hand hygiene
e) Minimising air-borne virus transmission
f) Minimising blood-borne virus transmission
g) Personal protective equipment
h) Waste segregation and disposal

1. An ultrasonic bath has failed a foil ablation test at the practice and requires servicing before it can be re-used. In the meantime, the staff are required to manually clean the dental instruments before they are sterilised. Which one of the options listed is the section of the IPC Policy that will provide the staff with the correct protocol to follow in this case?

2. During the summer holiday period the dental workplace has had to rely on a locum dentist to provide emergency cover to their patients, as the husband-and-wife owners are away together. On the first day of attendance the locum

dentist arrives wearing numerous bracelets and is informed by the practice manager that they cannot be worn while the dentist is treating patients. Which one of the options listed is the section of the IPC Policy that will corroborate the practice manager's advice?

3. A patient has undergone a clearance procedure before the fitting of a new upper full denture, and the dental nurse is left to clean the surgery after the patient has left. Several of the teeth were sound but periodontally involved, and others had failed old amalgam fillings present. The nurse is unsure whether the teeth can all be placed in the sharps box or not. Which one of the options listed is the section of the IPC Policy that will indicate the correct procedure to follow?

Topic: II

For each of the following infection prevention and control questions, select the single most appropriate answer from the option list. Each option might be used once, more than once or not at all.

a) B-type autoclave
b) Cleaning
c) Decontamination
d) Disinfection
e) Hand rub
f) Hand wash
g) N-type autoclave
h) Personal protective equipment
i) Sterilisation
j) Washer-disinfector

1. The safe re-processing of dental instruments involves the correct use of various items of equipment, ideally all located in a decontamination room that is separate from the clinical areas. Which one of the options listed is an item of equipment that is unsuitable for the sterilisation of hollow dental instruments, such as some items from an implant placement kit?

2. The World Health Organisation recommends all staff to follow the 'five moments of hand hygiene' to ensure that cross-infection in all healthcare settings is kept to a minimum. Which one of the options listed is a technique that can be used on dry hands to clean them between patients, where appropriate?

3. In line with the dental workplace's Infection Prevention and Control Policy, a staff member is carrying out the various validation tests required to ensure the correct working of the re-processing equipment. Which one of the options listed is the equipment item involved when a chemical dosing test is being carried out?

4. In line with the dental workplace's Infection Prevention and Control Policy, a staff member is carrying out the various validation tests required to ensure the correct working of the re-processing equipment. Which one of the options listed is the equipment item involved when a steam penetration test is being undertaken?

Topic: III

For each of the following infection prevention and control questions, select the single most appropriate answer from the option list. Each option might be used once, more than once or not at all.

a) Automatic control test
b) Blue mop
c) Distillation
d) DUWLs
e) PPE use
f) Protein residue test
g) Red mop
h) Reverse osmosis
i) Rinsing sink
j) Single-use items
k) Standard operating procedures
l) Standard precautions
m) Yellow mop

1. In line with guidance issued by the National Patient Safety Agency, cleaning equipment used to decontaminate the workplace environment should be colour-coded and only used in that colour's designated areas. This prevents the spread of micro-organism contamination from areas of high risk into areas of low risk. Which one of the options listed is the correct cleaning equipment to be used in the entrance foyer of the premises?

2. In line with current HTM 01-05 guidance, endodontic files and reamers may be decontaminated and re-used on the same patient, although they should be cleaned separately from other items before sterilisation. Which one of the options listed is a validation process for use with ultrasonic baths that will record the elimination of any pulp tissue from the instruments?

3. Dental treatment provision and the running of the dental workplace involves the use of copious amounts of water: to cool drills and scalers during treatment, in decontamination equipment and during cleaning activities. Which one of the options listed is the most likely area where biofilm contamination may occur from the water supply?

Answers

Multiple choice questions

1. *The correct answer is E.* These were previously referred to as 'universal precautions' and accommodate the fact that many patients may be unknown carriers of an infectious disease (such as Covid-19), where they show no symptoms of the disease but can transmit it to others. If all patients are assumed to be potential carriers and full infection prevention and control methods are carried out after every patient contact, the risk of cross-infection is massively reduced.

2. *The correct answer is E.* Autoclaves are also called sterilisers, as they apply high temperatures, pressure and sometimes a vacuum to their contents so that all micro-organisms and spores within the chamber are killed. The instruments are then safe to be used on another patient without the risk of transferring disease.

3. *The correct answer is A.* Cleaning involves the removal of visible debris from an item and may be achieved manually (using detergent solutions and brushes) or using an ultrasonic bath. The latter uses special chemicals in a tank that vibrates during use to dislodge debris from instruments.

4. *The correct answer is A.* Both products must be applied to the hands to carry out hand hygiene. The alcohol-based gel should be applied directly to dry hands and allowed to evaporate from the hands naturally, rather than being wiped dry. Water should not be mixed with the alcohol-based gel, whereas it must be used with the mild antibacterial liquid soap – before application and to rinse off once all areas of the hands have been cleaned. Wet hands must then be dried to avoid dry and cracked skin.

5. *The correct answer is E.* A visor, or face shield, is an impermeable plastic sheet held onto a head frame that covers the whole face from the forehead to below the chin, when worn correctly. No other options provide eye protection.

6. *The correct answer is D.* Special pre-made 'contaminated' sheets are available that are loaded into their holders and run through a washer-disinfector cycle. If the artificial contaminant has been sufficiently removed from the sheet at the end of the cycle, the machine has been shown to be working correctly.

7. *The correct answer is A.* Blue mop heads and handles, buckets, dustpans and brushes should be used in these areas only. They must not be used in any other areas of the workplace, such as surgeries, bathrooms, kitchens and decontamination areas.

8. *The correct answer is C.* The chlorine content of a bleach-based solution diminishes over time as the chlorine is lost from the solution as a gas, resulting in a gradually weaker solution. Hence the pungent smell of bleach products. Bleach-based solutions should therefore be made fresh each day.

9. *The correct answer is B.* The biocide chemical should always be present in the reservoir bottle system so that it is continually drawn through the hoses to the dental handpieces, scaler unit or triple syringe device during normal use. Some biocide manufacturers also recommend a regular 'shock' treatment is carried out (often monthly), where a more concentrated biocide solution is flushed through the DUWLs to ensure a biofilm build-up does not occur. The concentrated solution is then flushed out of the system before the equipment is used on a patient again.

10. *The correct answer is D.* Legionella bacteria can survive over a wide temperature range and will actively grow and expand as a colony between 20°C and 45°C. Consequently, cold water in the dental workplace should remain below 20°C and hot water should be maintained above 45°C.

11. *The correct answer is E.* The fourth stage of the washer-disinfector cycle is thermal disinfection, where the pre-set temperature and time are reached and maintained within the chamber. The temperature setting can be varied depending on the contents of the load to be disinfected – some items may be damaged by excessive temperatures.

12. *The correct answer is C.* Blood contains the protein haemoglobin, so a protein residue test will detect remaining contamination of instruments by blood if positive. After a cycle in the ultrasonic bath, items are rinsed and then wiped over with the test applicator. The applicator is then re-inserted into the test tube, where it reacts with an agent that changes colour if proteins are present. If there is no colour change, the items have been effectively cleaned of protein contamination.

13. *The correct answer is A.* The items can be returned to the clinical area for re-use that day only. If not re-used that day they must be re-processed and stored as for any of the other four options.

14. *The correct answer is C.* Used surgical items will be contaminated by a patient's blood and soft tissue debris so have the potential to transmit infection to others. They are categorised as hazardous infectious waste and should be disposed of in a sharps bin. Expired liner material, lead foil and study model casts are all categorised as non-hazardous waste, while X-ray fixer solution is categorised as hazardous chemical waste.

15. *The correct answer is E.* Covid-19, Hepatitis B and Influenza are all diseases caused by viruses, while Creutzfeld-Jakob disease is transmitted by prions.

16. *The correct answer is A.* The time, temperature and pressure parameters are the same for both types of autoclaves, but only the B-type are capable of producing a vacuum within the chamber during a sterilisation cycle.

Extended matching questions

Topic: I

1. *The correct answer is b).* This section of the IPC policy should detail the full decontamination process to be followed when re-processing instruments, including manual cleaning. Most dental workplaces clean instruments using an ultrasonic bath or a washer-disinfector rather than manually, but correct manual cleaning techniques must always be included in the IPC policy for exactly this scenario – where the automated technique cannot be used for whatever reason, so the staff must resort to the alternative manual technique.

2. *The correct answer is d).* Good hand hygiene is one of the most important methods of preventing the spread of infection, both in the clinical environment and generally. Hand jewellery such as rings and bracelets, when worn in the clinical environment, provide numerous tiny stagnation areas for micro-organisms and general debris contamination to gather and, unless scrubbed clean after treating each patient, they are very likely to be sources of cross-infection for the next patient.

3. *The correct answer is h).* The waste segregation section of the IPC policy should itemise the waste containers used in the workplace and which waste can be placed into each. The waste produced in the dental workplace will be categorised as non-hazardous, hazardous infectious or hazardous chemical waste. Sound teeth may be disposed of in the sharps bin, while teeth containing amalgam fillings should be disposed of as hazardous chemical waste.

Topic: II

1. *The correct answer is g).* N-type autoclaves are also called downward displacement autoclaves, and they sterilise items by drawing down super-heated steam over the chamber contents. The steam does not penetrate hollow items though, so contamination may still be present within their lumens after a sterilisation cycle.

2. *The correct answer is e).* Hand rubs are alcohol-based gels that can be used to disinfect the hands after removing PPE, between patients. The gel is applied to dry hands, not wet, and the cleaning routine is otherwise the same as for hand washing with soap and water.

3. *The correct answer is j).* This test is carried out to ensure that the detergent and/or disinfectant chemicals are released correctly into the machine during the operative cycle. It should also indicate when the level of either chemical is becoming low and requires replenishment.

4. *The correct answer is a).* B-type autoclaves are capable of producing a vacuum during an operative cycle, and this enables hollow items and items that have been packaged before sterilisation (such as surgical kits) to be sterilised. The steam penetration test is the method used to validate the correct action of

the machine during a vacuum cycle. A test strip placed into a helix holder should change colour in the presence of steam.

Topic: III

1. *The correct answer is b).* The entrance foyer of the workplace is classed as a communal area, where staff and patients simply enter and leave the premises. No clinical activities occur here and the area is not used as a bathroom or kitchen, so the correct colour code is blue.

2. *The correct answer is f).* Protein residue tests should be carried out weekly on the ultrasonic bath. After a cleaning and disinfection cycle has been completed, the instruments should be rinsed in distilled or reverse osmosis water and then wiped over with a test tip. The test tip is then inserted into a tube containing a chemical that changes colour if any protein residue is still present on the instruments. A photograph of the completed test tip can be taken and archived as evidence of a pass result, as the tips tend to continue changing colour over time and will eventually record a false-positive result.

3. *The correct answer is d).* Dental unit water lines (DUWLs) are the hoses that run from the bracket table to the dental handpieces, the three-in-one syringe and the scaler unit. Ideally, they should not be connected to the mains water supply directly and should use a reservoir bottle water supply instead. The bottle is filled from the distilled water or reverse osmosis supply within the workplace and changed daily. A specialist biocide chemical should also be present in the bottle every day.

8 General Anatomy and Physiology

Multiple choice questions

1. Dental nurses require an underpinning knowledge of various topics to enable them to understand specific dentally related subjects more readily. Which one of the following options is a topic concerned with how the body normally functions?
   A Anatomy
   B Biology
   C Medicine
   D Pathology
   E Physiology

2. The human body is a complex organism whose structure and function are studied to maintain health and to prevent or treat diseases. Which one of the following options is the correct term for various groups of tissues that perform related functions to each other?
   A Cells
   B Chromosomes
   C Nuclei
   D Organs
   E Systems

3. The human body has 10 systems that work together to maintain life and to allow the continuation of the species. Which one of the following options is the system concerned with the regulation and coordination of normal body functions by the secretion of hormones?
   A Digestive system
   B Endocrine system
   C Immune system
   D Nervous system
   E Reproductive system

Questions and Answers for Dental Nurses, Fourth Edition. Carole Hollins.

4. The heart is a muscular pumping organ situated towards the left side of the thoracic cavity. Which one of the following options is the most likely blood vessel through which the left atrium receives oxygenated blood from the capillary beds of the lungs?
   A Aorta
   B Inferior vena cava
   C Pulmonary artery
   D Pulmonary vein
   E Superior vena cava

5. When an artery passes over bone and the surrounding musculature, a patient's heartbeat can be determined and measured as their pulse rate. Which one of the following options is the pulse that can be detected at the inner surface of the elbow where the artery lies over the elbow joint?
   A Brachial pulse
   B Carotid pulse
   C Femoral pulse
   D Radial pulse
   E Temporal pulse

6. The circulatory system contains approximately 5 litres of blood in an adult and is composed of various cells floating in a specialised fluid. Which one of the following options is the element of blood responsible for helping to defend the body against attack by micro-organisms and disease?
   A Erythrocytes
   B Leucocytes
   C Plasma
   D Platelets
   E Thrombocytes

7. When completing a medical history form, patients are always asked to list all their medications so that they can receive safe and appropriate dental care. Which one of the following types of medication may be a cause for concern amongst the dental team when a patient attends for a surgical procedure to be carried out?
   A Analgesic
   B Antibiotic
   C Anticoagulant
   D Diuretic
   E Hormone-replacement

8. Throughout the body a gaseous exchange mechanism occurs within capillary beds, where oxygen is released into the surrounding tissues and replaced by carbon dioxide. Which one of the following options is the correct term for this mechanism?

A Dialysis
B Diastole
C External respiration
D Internal respiration
E Systole

9. The respiratory system has several protective mechanisms to ensure that it constantly functions to provide a clean and warm oxygen supply to the body tissues, without interruption. Which one of the following options is an anatomical feature that does not assist in this process?
A Cartilage lining of trachea
B Cilia
C Epiglottis
D Mucus coating
E Rich nasal blood supply

10. The digestive system is composed of various structures and organs that act together to digest food and fluids so that their components can be used by the body tissues to maintain life. Which one of the following options is the anatomical structure responsible for the reabsorption of water and salts into the body?
A Colon
B Liver
C Oesophagus
D Pancreas
E Stomach

11. The digestive system is composed of various structures and organs that act together to digest food and fluids so that their components can be used by the body tissues to maintain life. Which one of the following options is the anatomical structure responsible for releasing iron from any ingested food so that it can be used to produce new stocks of haemoglobin?
A Duodenum
B Ileum
C Liver
D Pancreas
E Stomach

12. The nervous system functions to allow us to experience consciousness and awareness of our surroundings and also to allow the regulation and coordination of body activities. Which one of the following options is the part of the system that allows us to smell and taste food products before digesting them?
A Autonomic nerves
B Enteric nerves
C Peripheral nerves

D Sensory organs
E Spinal cord

13. The nervous system functions to allow us to experience consciousness and awareness of our surroundings and also to allow the regulation and coordination of body activities. Which part of the system is responsible for transmitting impulses to the muscles of mastication to allow chewing movements to occur?
A Autonomic nerves
B Brain
C Enteric nerves
D Sensory nerves
E Somatic nerves

14. The brain lies within the bony structure of the skull and floats there bathed in cerebrospinal fluid. Which of the following options is the area of the brain that makes up the vast majority of the brain tissue itself?
A Cerebellum
B Cerebrum
C Corpus callosum
D Medulla oblongata
E Pons

15. The nerves supplying the head and neck region leave the brain directly from its under-surface through various natural bony openings of the skull as the 12 pairs of cranial nerves. Which one of the following options is the cranial nerve composed of motor fibres only, which effect movement of the tongue muscles when stimulated?
A Facial nerve
B Glossopharyngeal nerve
C Hypoglossal nerve
D Optic nerve
E Trigeminal nerve

16. The nerves supplying the head and neck region leave the brain directly from its under-surface through various natural bony openings of the skull as the 12 pairs of cranial nerves. Which one of the following options is the cranial nerve that is partially composed of sensory nerves that transmit pressure sensations from the teeth to the brain?
A Facial nerve
B Glossopharyngeal nerve
C Hypoglossal nerve
D Optic nerve
E Trigeminal nerve

17. The nerves supplying the head and neck region leave the brain directly from its under-surface through various natural bony openings of the skull as the 12 pairs of cranial nerves. Which one of the following options is the cranial nerve that contains a motor component that effects swallowing movements by stimulating the muscles of the oropharynx?
    - A Facial nerve
    - B Glossopharyngeal nerve
    - C Hypoglossal nerve
    - D Optic nerve
    - E Trigeminal nerve

18. The nerves supplying the head and neck region leave the brain directly from its under-surface through various natural bony openings of the skull as the 12 pairs of cranial nerves. Which one of the following options are the two pairs of cranial nerves that transmit all taste sensations from the tongue to the brain?
    - A Facial and glossopharyngeal nerves
    - B Facial and trigeminal nerves
    - C Glossopharyngeal and hypoglossal nerves
    - D Hypoglossal and facial nerves
    - E Trigeminal and hypoglossal nerves

Extended matching questions

For each of the following general anatomy questions, select the single most appropriate answer from the option list. Each option might be used once, more than once or not at all.

a) Aorta
b) Cerebellum
c) Cerebrum
d) Diaphragm
e) Epiglottis
f) Gallbladder
g) Left ventricle
h) Liver
i) Motor nerves
j) Pancreas
k) Pulmonary vein
l) Right atrium
m) Sensory nerves
n) Superior vena cava
o) Trachea

1. The heart is a muscular pumping organ that is responsible for transporting blood around the whole body. It is formed of two sides that usually do not communicate with each other, with two chambers in each side. Which one of the options listed is the chamber that pumps oxygenated blood out to the body?

2. The nervous system is composed of the brain, spinal cord and billions of cranial and peripheral neurones. Which one of the options listed is the type of neurone that carries information from the body to the brain to be interpreted and acted upon?

3. The digestive system acts to break down the food we eat and release the various chemical components to be used by the body tissues to create energy. Which one of the options listed is the digestive organ responsible for the storage of vitamins released from digested foods?

4. The respiratory system is responsible for taking in oxygen from the atmosphere and removing carbon dioxide from the body tissues. Which one of the options listed is the muscular sheet that separates the respiratory system in the thorax from the digestive system in the abdomen?

Answers

Multiple choice questions

1. *The correct answer is E.* This topic is the branch of biology that studies the functions and activities of the organs, tissues and cells of the body, and the physical and chemical way in which they interact to maintain the life of the organism.

2. *The correct answer is E.* So, for example, the various tissues that make up the components of the digestive system are all concerned with extracting chemicals and nutrients from the food we eat, to be used throughout the body for growth and repair.

3. *The correct answer is B.* The endocrine system is composed of all glands that secrete hormones directly into the circulatory system, to be transported around the body to their area of need.

4. *The correct answer is D.* By definition, veins are the blood vessels that carry deoxygenated blood away from an organ – in this case, the lungs. However, reoxygenation of blood occurs in the lungs so the vessels carrying blood away from them, the pair of pulmonary veins (one from each lung), actually carry oxygenated blood and are the only major veins in the body to do so. The oxygenated blood is received by the left atrium and travels through the left side of the heart before being pumped out and around the body.

5. *The correct answer is A.* The brachial artery lies in this position, and in a thinner person with normal musculature the artery can be seen to be pulsing when the arm is held straight out with the inner surface uppermost.

6. *The correct answer is B.* Leucocytes are a group of white blood cells that are made in several areas of the immune system, such as the lymph nodes and bone marrow, and constantly circulate throughout the body in the bloodstream. When a micro-organism attack occurs, massive numbers of leucocytes are produced and transported to the area to fight them off – often resulting in the tell-tale sign of 'swollen glands' (lymph nodes) that indicates a person has an infection.

7. *The correct answer is C.* Anticoagulants are prescribed to prevent the formation of a blood clot that may result in a stroke or a heart attack for susceptible patients. However, they may also prevent adequate blood clotting following trauma or surgery, so patients prescribed these medications should be treated with great caution by the dental team, to ensure that their dental care is provided safely.

8. *The correct answer is D.* The released oxygen is used by the surrounding tissues to work and carry out their functions, producing the waste product carbon dioxide, which is carried away in the bloodstream to the lungs, where it is exhaled.

9. *The correct answer is C.* The epiglottis is a cartilage flap in the larynx that closes off the trachea during swallowing, so that food or fluids are directed into the digestive system via the oesophagus. It plays no role in the act of respiration. All of the other options are protective mechanisms that ensure the respiratory system is held open to the atmosphere, and the air inhaled is both clean and warm so that the lungs are not irritated during inspiration.

10. *The correct answer is A.* In addition, the large intestines (colon) store digestive waste products before they are eliminated as faeces.

11. *The correct answer is E.* The acid and enzymes released by the stomach cells act on foods containing iron to release it. The iron is then stored by the liver before being distributed as required to produce haemoglobin. This is then carried around the body in the red blood cells.

12. *The correct answer is D.* The sensory organs are the eyes, ears, nose and tongue and the latter two allow for the sensations of smell and taste to occur.

13. *The correct answer is E.* Somatic nerves are motor nerves that carry impulses from the brain to the musculoskeletal system to allow voluntary movement of the relevant part of the body. The movements produced are controlled by conscious thought (voluntary) and occur due to the coordinated contraction and relaxation of the relevant muscle groups involved.

14. *The correct answer is B.* The cerebrum forms the two cerebral hemispheres (left and right) of grey matter that make up the majority of the brain. They appear as vastly convoluted folds of specialised nerve tissue responsible for the mental processes of thought, learning, memory and understanding.

15. *The correct answer is C.* All of the other options are sensory nerves or have sensory and autonomic components present too.

16. *The correct answer is E.* The trigeminal nerve is that of most interest to the dental team, as it transmits sensations from the whole oral cavity to the brain, in addition to effecting the movements of the muscles of mastication.

17. *The correct answer is B.* The glossopharyngeal nerve also has a sensory component that transmits taste sensations from the back of the tongue to the brain and an autonomic component that stimulates saliva secretions from the submandibular and sublingual salivary glands.

18. *The correct answer is A.* The sensory components of these nerves transmit taste sensations from the front part of the tongue and the back of the tongue to the brain, respectively.

Extended matching questions

1. *The correct answer is g).* The left atrium receives oxygenated blood from the lungs and passes it through to the left ventricle from where it is pumped out to the body via the aorta.
2. *The correct answer is m).* Sensory nerves transmit sensations from the body to the brain, such as pain, temperature, touch and the specialised sensations of sight, sound, taste and smell.
3. *The correct answer is h).* The liver acts as the chemical factory of the body and receives nutrient-rich blood from the stomach and intestines via the portal vein. The liver stores these nutrients (including vitamins) until they are required by the body cells.
4. *The correct answer is d).* The diaphragm forms the base of the thorax and the top of the abdominal cavity, separating the two cavities except for the point where the oesophagus passes through it to reach the stomach. The contraction of the diaphragm downwards during inhalation helps to increase the size of the thorax so that the lungs expand and fill with air. When it relaxes, the air is forced back out of the lungs during exhalation.

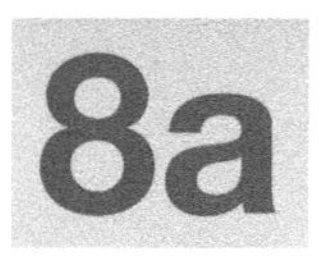

Head and Neck Anatomy and Physiology

Multiple choice questions

1. The cranium is made up of eight bony plates that enclose the brain like a helmet and fit together tightly at the coronoid sutures. Which one of the following options is the bony plate that has a large hole called the foramen magnum present, through which the spinal cord exits the base of the brain and enters the vertebral column?
   A Ethmoid
   B Occipital
   C Parietal
   D Sphenoid
   E Temporal

2. The face forms the middle section of the skull and is composed of 11 bones joined together at various sutures and contains the sensory organs of the eyes and nose. Which one of the following options is the facial bone that articulates with the temporal bone posteriorly and the maxilla anteriorly to form the cheekbones?
   A Lacrimal bone
   B Nasal bone
   C Palatine bone
   D Vomer
   E Zygomatic bone

3. The maxilla forms the middle third of the facial region of the skull and is composed of two hollow bones joined together in the midline. Which one of the following options is the correct term for this hollow cavity?
   A Antrum
   B Nose
   C Orbit
   D Oropharynx
   E Soft palate

4. The lower jaw is called the mandible and is the only bone of the skull that has a moveable joint articulation with its surrounding bones. Which one of the following options is the anatomical structure of the mandible that articulates with the temporal bone of the skull?
   A Coronoid process
   B Head of condyle
   C Lingula
   D Ramus
   E Sigmoid notch

5. Many of the bones of the skull contain natural bony openings (foramina) to allow the passage of nerves and blood vessels to the tissues of the head and neck region. Which one of the following options is the name of the foramen through which the inferior dental nerve exits the mandible?
   A Greater palatine foramen
   B Incisive foramen
   C Mandibular foramen
   D Mental foramen
   E Supraorbital foramen

6. The temporomandibular joint is the hinge joint between the cranium and the mandible, and its articulation between the temporal bone and the condylar head allows the lower jaw to open and close. When the condylar head moves too far forwards it may become stuck in front of the articular eminence. Which one of the following options is the correct term for this occurrence?
   A Bruxism
   B Dislocation
   C Fracture
   D Subluxation
   E Trismus

7. The muscles of mastication are four sets of muscles connected between the mandible and the base of the cranium or the face, whose contractions allow chewing movements and mouth closure to occur. Which one of the following options is the muscle that runs from the cranium to the coronoid process of the mandible and acts to pull the mandible backwards and closed?
   A Buccinator
   B Lateral pterygoid
   C Masseter
   D Medial pterygoid
   E Temporalis

8. The suprahyoid muscles lie beneath the mandible in the neck and act to assist in swallowing movements and mouth opening. Which one of the following options is the muscle that runs from the hyoid bone in the throat to the inner surface of the mental symphysis of the mandible?

A Anterior digastric
B Buccinator
C Geniohyoid
D Mylohyoid
E Orbicularis oris

9. The three groups of muscles of the head and neck region that are relevant to the dental team are those of mastication, suprahyoids and facial expression. Which one of the following options is the muscle that is a member of the latter group and assists in enabling speech to occur by movement of the lips?
A Anterior digastric
B Buccinator
C Masseter
D Mylohyoid
E Orbicularis oris

10. The head and neck are innervated by 12 pairs of cranial nerves, and several of these nerves are a combination of both motor and sensory fibres. Which one of the following options is the cranial nerve that consists only of motor fibres that effect movement of the tongue muscles to allow speech and assist in the breakdown of ingested food before moving it to the pharynx for swallowing?
A Facial nerve
B Glossopharyngeal nerve
C Hypoglossal nerve
D Optic nerve
E Trigeminal nerve

11. The trigeminal nerve (fifth cranial nerve) splits into three divisions before leaving the cranium, one of which is the maxillary division. Which one of the following options is the branch of the maxillary nerve that emerges from the base of the orbital cavity and transmits touch sensation from the labial gingivae of the upper incisor and canine teeth to the brain?
A Anterior superior dental nerve
B Greater palatine nerve
C Middle superior dental nerve
D Nasopalatine nerve
E Posterior superior dental nerve

12. The trigeminal nerve (fifth cranial nerve) splits into three divisions before leaving the cranium, one of which is the mandibular division. Which one of the following options is the branch of the mandibular nerve that crosses over the external oblique ridge and transmits touch sensation from the buccal gingivae of the lower molar teeth?
A Inferior dental nerve
B Lingual nerve
C Long buccal nerve

D Mental nerve
E Muscular branch

13. The head and neck regions of the body are supplied with oxygenated blood via the internal and external carotid arteries. Which one of the following options is the blood vessel that the carotid arteries branch from before travelling to the head and neck regions?
A Aorta
B Inferior vena cava
C Pulmonary artery
D Pulmonary vein
E Superior vena cava

14. Deoxygenated blood is removed from the head and neck regions of the body via the internal and external jugular veins. Which one of the following options is the blood vessel that the jugular veins drain into, so that the blood can be reoxygenated in the lungs?
A Aorta
B Inferior vena cava
C Pulmonary artery
D Pulmonary vein
E Superior vena cava

15. The trigeminal nerve (fifth cranial nerve) splits into three divisions before leaving the cranium, one of which is the maxillary division. Which one of the following options is the branch of the maxillary nerve that splits off in the floor of the orbital cavity and passes down the walls of the maxillary antrum to transmit pain sensation from the upper premolar teeth to the brain?
A Anterior superior dental nerve
B Greater palatine nerve
C Middle superior dental nerve
D Nasopalatine nerve
E Posterior superior dental nerve

16. The head and neck are innervated by 12 pairs of cranial nerves, and several of these nerves are a combination of both motor and sensory fibres. Which one of the following options is the cranial nerve that consists of sensory fibres from the facial soft tissues and motor fibres that supply some of the suprahyoids and the muscles of mastication?
A Facial nerve
B Glossopharyngeal nerve
C Hypoglossal nerve
D Optic nerve
E Trigeminal nerve

17. The muscles of mastication are four sets of muscles connected between the mandible and the base of the cranium or the face, whose contractions allow chewing movements and mouth closure to occur. Which one of the following options is the muscle that runs from the cranium to the inner surface of the mandibular ramus and angle and acts to close the mandible?
    A Buccinator
    B Lateral pterygoid
    C Masseter
    D Medial pterygoid
    E Temporalis

18. Abnormal or parafunctional habits of a patient, such as clenching and grinding the teeth over a long period (bruxing), are common findings by the dental team during oral examination. Which one of the following options are signs or symptoms that are unlikely to indicate that a patient performs these bruxing movements?
    A Erosion
    B Facial pain
    C Fractured fillings
    D Sore tongue
    E Trismus

Extended matching questions

For each of the following head and neck anatomy and physiology questions, select the single most appropriate answer from the option list. Each option might be used once, more than once or not at all.

a) Facial nerve
b) Glenoid fossa
c) Greater palatine nerve
d) Incisive foramen
e) Lateral pterygoid
f) Mandibular foramen
g) Masseter
h) Maxilla
i) Middle superior dental nerve
j) Sphenoid bone
k) Temporal bone

1. The muscles of mastication are those running between the skull and the mandible that are responsible for closing the mouth and chewing movements. Which one of the options listed is the muscle of mastication running between the zygomatic arch and the mandible?

2. The temporomandibular joint is the only moveable joint in the head region and is formed between the head of the mandibular condyle and the temporal bone at the base of the skull. Which one of the options listed is the area of the temporal bone where the head of condyle rests when the jaw is closed?

3. The nerve supply to the head is extensive and supplied by the 12 pairs of cranial nerves, which leave the brain directly through the base of the skull to innervate the area. Which one of the options listed is the name of the seventh cranial nerve that supplies some taste sensation from the tongue?

4. The trigeminal nerve is the cranial nerve that supplies some facial soft tissues, the teeth and their soft tissues and the muscles of mastication. Which one of the options listed is the point where a branch of its maxillary division passes through the floor of the nose onto the palate to supply sensation from the palatal gingivae of the incisors to the brain?

Answers

Multiple choice questions

1. *The correct answer is B.* The occipital bone is a single plate lying at the back and partial underside of the cranium. The nobbled projections felt along its lower edge allow for muscular attachments and enable the head to be lifted up.
2. *The correct answer is E.* The cheekbones are correctly termed the zygomatic arches.
3. *The correct answer is A.* The two maxillary antra, or sinuses, lie to the sides of and are connected to the nasal cavity. They are normally air-filled but will contain mucus and debris if they become infected by bacteria or viruses, such as when someone suffers a common cold.
4. *The correct answer is B.* The head of condyle is the rounded projection of bone at the back of the vertical section of the mandible, the ramus. It forms a hinge joint with the temporal bone of the cranium, where the condyle sits in the glenoid fossa. Articulation of the joint allows the mandible to open and close, swing from side to side, and move forwards so the teeth sit in an edge-to-edge position.
5. *The correct answer is D.* The inferior dental nerve enters the mandible through the mandibular foramen on the inner surface of the ramus and exits the bone through the mental foramen, which lies on the outer surface of the body between the roots of the lower premolar teeth.
6. *The correct answer is B.* The joint is said to be dislocated and will require manual manipulation to relocate the condylar head into the glenoid fossa. This often has to be carried out under sedation or general anaesthetic, so that the muscles of mastication around the joint are sufficiently relaxed to enable the mandible to be manipulated.
7. *The correct answer is E.* The temporal muscle runs from the temporal bone of the cranium, under the zygomatic arch to the coronoid process of the mandible.
8. *The correct answer is A.* The digastric muscle has an anterior and posterior belly, and only the former is of relevance to the dental nurse. It is innervated by the motor branch of the trigeminal nerve and acts to lift the hyoid bone and larynx during swallowing and pulls the mandible down to open the mouth.
9. *The correct answer is E.* This is a ring of tissue surrounding the oral aperture that connects to several other muscles of facial expression within the soft tissues of the face. Their various muscular actions together allow the mouth to perform many actions, such as some speech sounds, smiling, pursing, whistling and so on.

10. *The correct answer is C.* The hypoglossal nerve (12th cranial nerve) effects the muscles of the mobile anterior section of the tongue, allowing it to perform various movements.

11. *The correct answer is A.* This branch also transmits sensation from these teeth to the brain.

12. *The correct answer is C.* The long buccal nerve splits from the mandibular nerve before the inferior dental component enters the mandible at the mandibular foramen, on the inner surface of the ramus.

13. *The correct answer is A.* The aorta leaves the left ventricle as the main artery in the body, and the common carotid arteries are the first branches from the arch of the aorta. The common carotid arteries split into the external and internal branches at the top of the neck, with the internal branches then travelling into the cranium itself.

14. *The correct answer is E.* The superior vena cava is the main vein collecting deoxygenated blood from structures above the heart, to transport it to the right atrium, the right ventricle and then to the lungs for reoxygenation via the pulmonary arteries.

15. *The correct answer is C.* This nerve also transmits sensations from the anterior half of the upper first molar teeth and the buccal gingivae of these teeth and the upper premolars.

16. *The correct answer is E.* The trigeminal nerve (fifth cranial nerve) has three divisions – the ophthalmic, the maxillary and the mandibular. All three contain sensory fibres from the face and jaws, including the teeth, while the mandibular division also effects muscular movement of the jaws.

17. *The correct answer is D.* This muscle originates from the medial pterygoid plate at the base of the cranium and runs forwards to insert onto the inner surface of the mandible.

18. *The correct answer is A.* Erosion of the teeth is caused by exposure to acids, either in the diet or due to repeated reflux of the acidic contents of the stomach. When patients habitually clench and grind their teeth, they will exhibit tooth attrition.

Extended matching questions

1. *The correct answer is g).* Masseter originates on the outer surface of the zygomatic arch (cheekbone) and inserts on the outer surface of the mandibular ramus and angle. On contraction it closes the mandible.

2. *The correct answer is b).* The glenoid fossa is a hollowed region of the temporal bone with a raised ridge anteriorly called the articular eminence. During

jaw movements, if the head of condyle slips out of the fossa and past the articular eminence, the jaw becomes dislocated.

3. *The correct answer is a).* The facial nerve is a combination nerve, carrying both sensory and motor fibres. Its sensory component carries taste sensation from the front of the tongue, and its motor component supplies the muscles of facial expression and the secretory action of the submandibular and sublingual salivary glands.

4. *The correct answer is d).* The nasopalatine nerve carries sensation from this area, through the incisive foramen into the floor of the nose and back to the brain. The nerve was previously called the long sphenopalatine in recognition of its extensive length, running from the front of the palate to the brain.

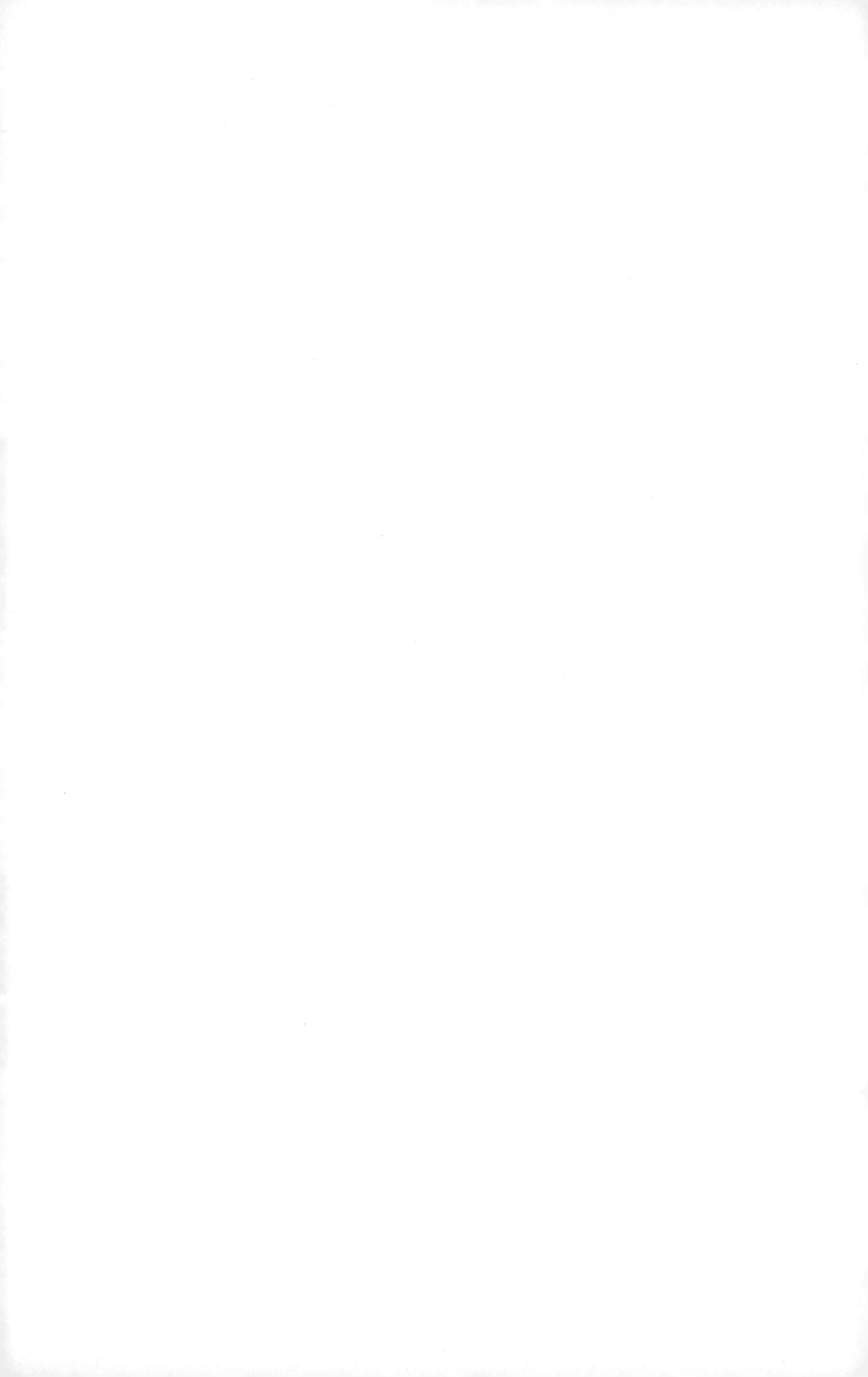

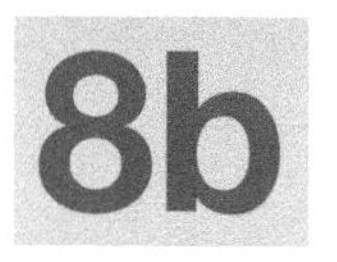

8b Oral Anatomy and Physiology

Multiple choice questions

1. There are several distinct types of mucous membrane found in various areas of the oral cavity. Which one of the following options is an area that is not covered by that called the masticatory membrane?
   A Dorsum of the tongue
   B Floor of the mouth
   C Gingivae
   D Hard palate
   E Sides of the tongue

2. There are many anatomical structures within the oral cavity, all with varying functions. Which one of the following options is a structure that functions to seal off the oral cavity from the nasal cavity during the act of swallowing, to prevent food and fluids passing into the nose?
   A Labial sulcus
   B Oropharynx
   C Soft palate
   D Tonsil
   E Uvula

3. The act of swallowing is a complicated one, involving many muscles and structures within the oral cavity and the throat. Which one of the following options is the structure that is responsible for preventing the food bolus from passing into the trachea during swallowing?
   A Body of tongue
   B Epiglottis
   C Larynx
   D Soft palate
   E Uvula

Questions and Answers for Dental Nurses, Fourth Edition. Carole Hollins.

4. Several diseases and disorders can affect the structures of the oral cavity so that they cannot perform their normal functions correctly. Which one of the following options is the term used to describe the condition of having a reduced salivary flow, making normal acts such as swallowing difficult for the sufferer to achieve?
   A Dysphagia
   B Glossitis
   C Laryngitis
   D Ptyalism
   E Xerostomia

5. Several diseases and disorders can affect the structures of the oral cavity so that they cannot perform their normal functions correctly. Which one of the following options is the term used to describe the condition of having a sore and inflamed tongue, with the dorsum of the organ appearing smooth and glazed?
   A Dysphagia
   B Glossitis
   C Laryngitis
   D Ptyalism
   E Xerostomia

6. The teeth are the anatomical structures within the oral cavity that are of the greatest relevance to the dental team. Which one of the following options is the correct term used to name each surface of a tooth in its relationship to the midline of the jaw and its surrounding anatomy, enabling a patient's dentition to be charted accurately?
   A Eruption
   B Exfoliation
   C Impaction
   D Morphology
   E Nomenclature

7. All teeth are composed of the same four tissues – enamel, dentine, cementum and pulp. Which one of the following options is a description of the layout of dentine tissue?
   A Calcium hydroxyapatite crystals
   B Fluorapatite crystals
   C Hollow tubes
   D Interprismatic substance
   E Prisms

8. Which one of the following options is a feature found in enamel, dentine and cementum but not the pulp?
   A Calcium hydroxyapatite crystals
   B Fluorapatite crystals
   C Hollow tubes

D Interprismatic substance
E Prisms

9. All teeth consist of various tissues that contain both organic and inorganic components. Which one of the following options is the tooth tissue composed of 80% calcium hydroxyapatite crystals and that forms the bulk of the tooth and root?
   A Cementum
   B Dentine
   C Enamel
   D Pulp
   E Secondary dentine

10. Each surface of every tooth has its own name in relation to the midline of each jaw and the anatomical structures surrounding it – a system called tooth surface nomenclature. Which one of the following options is the term used to describe the biting surface of all posterior teeth?
    A Cervical
    B Incisal
    C Labial
    D Occlusal
    E Palatal

11. The human dentition consists of a set of both primary and secondary teeth that have no ability to grow once they are fully formed. Which one of the following options is a feature of both primary and secondary second lower molars?
    A Cusp of Carabelli
    B Divergent roots
    C Large pulp chamber
    D Thick enamel
    E Two roots

12. Teeth can be identified by the number of cusps and roots that they have, whether still in the oral cavity (by radiography) or after extraction. Which one of the following options is a tooth that normally has two roots and four cusps?
    A Lower deciduous canine
    B Lower deciduous first molar
    C Lower first premolar
    D Upper first premolar
    E Upper permanent canine

13. Teeth can be identified by the number of cusps and roots that they have, whether still in the oral cavity (by radiography) or after extraction. Which one of the following options are a pair of teeth that normally both have three roots and five cusps?
    A Upper 6 and upper 7
    B Upper D and upper 7

C Upper D and upper E
D Upper E and upper 6
E Upper E and upper 7

14. The teeth forming both the primary and secondary dentitions tend to erupt within a given time period, referred to as their average eruption dates. Which one of the following options is the secondary tooth that erupts around age 6 to 7 years and is normally the main chewing tooth in the dental arch?
A Lower first molar
B Lower second premolar
C Upper canine
D Upper central incisor
E Upper second molar

15. The secondary dentition normally has eight teeth in each quadrant, assuming none are congenitally missing. Which one of the following options is a tooth that is used to pierce and tear food and has a cingulum?
A Lower canine
B Lower first premolar
C Lower second premolar
D Upper first molar
E Upper second premolar

16. The supporting structures of the teeth are collectively referred to as the periodontium and function to hold the teeth in their sockets. Which one of the following options is a tissue that is not found in the periodontium?
A Alveolar bone
B Cementum
C Gingiva
D Periodontal ligament
E Radicular pulp

17. The gingiva is one of the supporting structures of the teeth, collectively referred to as the periodontium. Which one of the following options is the type of gingival tissue present at the point where the tooth and the periodontium attach to each other?
A Attached gingiva
B Junctional epithelium
C Marginal gingiva
D Mucoperiosteum
E Sulcular epithelium

18. The periodontium is the collective term used for the supporting structures of the teeth that hold them in their sockets, one of which is the gingiva. Which one of the following options is the tissue that lines the inner surface of the shallow space surrounding each tooth, the gingival crevice?

A Attached gingiva
B Junctional epithelium
C Marginal gingiva
D Mucoperiosteum
E Sulcular epithelium

19. The periodontal ligament is a specialised fibrous tissue that attaches the teeth to the surrounding gingivae and alveolar bone. It is composed of groups of fibres that run in various directions between these structures. Which one of the following options is the group of fibres that run between the bone and most of the root length and help to prevent tooth rotation and intrusion?
A Apical fibres
B Free gingival fibres
C Horizontal fibres
D Oblique fibres
E Transeptal fibres

20. The salivary glands are present around the oral cavity as one of the three pairs of major glands, or within the mucosal lining of the oral cavity as one of numerous minor glands. Which one of the following options is a feature of the major salivary glands, the parotids?
A Are endocrine glands
B Innervated by the facial nerve
C Lie below the mylohyoid line
D Most likely to develop benign tumours
E Secrete via the Wharton ducts

21. The salivary glands are present around the oral cavity as one of the three pairs of major glands or within the mucosal lining of the oral cavity as one of numerous minor glands. Which one of the following options is a feature of the major salivary glands, the sublinguals?
A Innervated by the glossopharyngeal nerve
B Lie above the mylohyoid line
C Most likely to develop malignant tumours
D Most likely to develop salivary calculi
E Secrete via the Wharton ducts

22. Saliva is the watery fluid produced in the salivary glands and secreted into the oral cavity, and it contains many different components. Which one of the following options is the saliva component that acts to promote wound healing in the oral cavity?
A Antibodies
B Leucocytes
C Mucus
D Salivary amylase
E Water

Extended matching questions

For each of the following oral anatomy and physiology questions, select the single most appropriate answer from the option list. Each option might be used once, more than once or not at all.

a) Ameloblasts
b) Apical foramen
c) Cementum
d) Dentine
e) Enamel
f) Fibrils
g) Hollow tubes
h) Interprismatic substance
i) Odontoblasts
j) Prisms
k) Pulp

1. Microscopically teeth are composed of four distinct layers, all but one of which is made up mainly of inorganic calcium hydroxyapatite crystals. Which one of the options listed is the layer that can incorporate fluoride into its crystalline structure, so making the tooth stronger and more able to resist acid attacks?
2. The dentine layer forms the bulk of each tooth throughout the crown and root sections and is the layer where dental caries can invade the tooth structure most readily. During a carious attack, the tooth attempts to protect the pulp by laying down a layer of secondary dentine over the pulp chamber. Which one of the options listed is the cell type involved in the laying down of secondary dentine?
3. The dentine layer contains the end sections of the sensory nerves that innervate the teeth, transmitting temperature and pain sensations accordingly. Which one of the options listed is the term used to describe these nerve end sections, as they occur within the dentine?
4. The enamel layer forms the outermost layer of the crown of each tooth and is composed mainly of inorganic calcium hydroxyapatite crystals. Which one of the options listed is the term used to describe the organic matrix within which these crystals lie?

Answers

Multiple choice questions

1. *The correct answer is B.* The floor of the mouth is covered by lining membrane that provides a physical barrier between anything within the oral cavity and its deeper structures.
2. *The correct answer is C.* The soft palate is a flap of soft tissue attached to the back of the hard palate.
3. *The correct answer is B.* The epiglottis is a flap of cartilage lying in the throat at the top of the trachea, which it falls across to seal during the act of swallowing. This action guides the food bolus away from the trachea and into the oesophagus, where it passes on its journey to the stomach.
4. *The correct answer is E.* Although having a dry mouth occasionally due to anxiety or mouth breathing, a persistent reduction in salivary flow is correctly termed xerostomia. It may occur due to conditions such as Sjogren's syndrome or following radiotherapy for cancer affecting the head or neck tissues.
5. *The correct answer is B.* This condition may occur due to anaemia, vitamin B deficiency or a hormonal disturbance such as pregnancy.
6. *The correct answer is E.* Each surface of a tooth is designated a descriptive name using this terminology as described, so that all dental personnel have an accurate description of the dentition. Examples include the terms mesial, incisal, buccal, palatal and so on.
7. *The correct answer is C.* The hollow tubes of dentine contain sensory nerve fibrils that transmit hot and cold sensations from the pulp to the brain.
8. *The correct answer is A.* The pulp is not a calcified tissue and therefore contains no mineral crystals and is composed purely of soft tissue.
9. *The correct answer is B.* Dentine forms the inner layer of tissue of every tooth, lying beneath the enamel of the crown and the cementum of the root.
10. *The correct answer is D.* The term applies in both arches and to all premolar and molar teeth.
11. *The correct answer is E.* Primary second lower molars have divergent roots and a large pulp chamber, secondary second lower molars have thick enamel and neither second molars have a cusp of Carabelli.
12. *The correct answer is B.* Only molar teeth have more than two cusps.
13. *The correct answer is D.* Each is the largest tooth of the upper arch in the primary and secondary dentition, respectively.
14. *The correct answer is A.* Lower and upper first permanent molars usually begin erupting at a similar time to the lower permanent central incisors. Anecdotally, the lower permanent first molars appear as the most heavily

restored teeth in many patients' dentition, as they erupt so early and are often the main chewing teeth so undergo the most chewing use.

15. *The correct answer is A.* Incisors and canines have a raised area on their lingual or palatal surface that is called a cingulum.

16. *The correct answer is E.* The pulp supplies blood to the tooth and transmits sensations from it to the brain but plays no part in holding the tooth in its socket.

17. *The correct answer is B.* This is a specialised gingival tissue within the gingival crevice that forms an anatomical junction between the teeth and the rest of the oral cavity, providing a mechanical barrier between the two areas.

18. *The correct answer is E.* The gingival crevice is also referred to as the gingival sulcus, hence sulcular epithelium. The junctional epithelium is only present within the sulcus at the point where the gingiva attaches to the tooth.

19. *The correct answer is D.* Oblique fibres run at an angle from the alveolar bone down to the cementum of the root, from just below the bony crest to just above the root apex.

20. *The correct answer is D.* The parotids are the major glands most likely to develop both benign and malignant tumours.

21. *The correct answer is B.* The sublingual glands lie above the mylohyoid line in the front area of the floor of the mouth.

22. *The correct answer is A.* In particular, immunoglobulin A is present in saliva and helps to promote wound healing. Leucocytes (white blood cells) are present when required and act as a defence mechanism against oral infection and disease.

Extended matching questions

1. *The correct answer is e).* Enamel forms the outer layer of each tooth and is a non-living tissue, as it does not contain nerves or blood vessels. Consequently, enamel cannot grow and repair itself, but it can change chemically when exposed to fluoride.

2. *The correct answer is i).* Odontoblasts are the cells that form dentine during tooth formation and are present throughout life as a layer of cells lying along the inner edge of the pulp chamber, where they form more dentine as necessary.

3. *The correct answer is f).* The fibrils lie in the hollow tube structure of dentine and are extensions of the nerve tissue within the pulp chamber.

4. *The correct answer is h).* Interprismatic substance is the organic matrix within which the inorganic crystalline prisms lie. It makes up just 4% of the structure of enamel.

9 Dental Pathology and Microbiology

Multiple choice questions

1. Many diseases are caused by contamination of the body cells by microscopic living organisms, collectively called pathogenic micro-organisms, or pathogens. Which one of the following options are pathogens that are single-celled organisms and can cause disease?
   A Bacteria
   B Fungi
   C Prions
   D Protozoa
   E Viruses

2. The dental team may potentially be exposed to many pathogenic micro-organisms while carrying out their routine actions to care for the oral health of their patients. Which one of the following options is a group of chemicals that are especially useful in destroying bacterial contamination of hard surfaces in the surgery?
   A Antibiotics
   B Antifungals
   C Bactericides
   D Vaccines
   E Viricides

3. Although viruses are not associated with dental caries or periodontal disease, they are of importance to the dental team in relation to infection prevention and control. Which one of the following options is a virus that is responsible for some cases of oropharyngeal cancer?
   A Epstein-Barr
   B Hepatitis B
   C Herpes varicella
   D Human papillomavirus
   E Paramyxovirus

Questions and Answers for Dental Nurses, Fourth Edition. Carole Hollins.

4. Although viruses are not associated with dental caries or periodontal disease, they are of importance to the dental team in relation to infection prevention and control. Which one of the following options is the virus responsible for chickenpox, a viral infection that often affects the areas of the face supplied by the trigeminal nerve?
   A Coxsackievirus
   B Herpes simplex
   C Herpes varicella
   D Herpes zoster
   E Human immunodeficiency virus

5. Many diseases occur as the result of fungal infections of the skin and mucous membranes, including the soft tissues that line the oral cavity. Which one of the following options is a micro-organism that is associated with several fungal disorders that can occur in the mouth?
   A *Borrelia vincenti*
   B *Campylobacter rectus*
   C *Candida albicans*
   D *Porphyromonas gingivalis*
   E *Staphylococcus aureus*

6. Tissue damage, illness and disease can occur to body cells from a variety of sources, besides that of attack by a pathogenic micro-organism. Which one of the following options is a lesion most likely to be caused by an uncontrolled and abnormal overgrowth of the body cells?
   A Cyst
   B Infection
   C Inflammation
   D Tumour
   E Ulcer

7. Dental pathology is the study of diseases and conditions that specifically affect the oral cavity and their effects on its hard and soft tissues. Which one of the following options is a lesion that is caused by a bacterial infection of a tooth?
   A Apthous ulcer
   B Candidosis
   C Caries
   D Leukoplakia
   E Stomatitis

8. Dental pathology is the study of diseases and conditions that specifically affect the oral cavity and their effects on its hard and soft tissues. Which one of the following options is the term used to describe the presence of a white patch that cannot be removed from the oral mucosa by wiping?
   A Apthous ulcer
   B Candidosis
   C Caries

D Leukoplakia
E Stomatitis

9. When any body tissues are exposed to physical or chemical irritants (such as fire or acids) or are breached by pathogenic micro-organisms, the tissues affected undergo an inflammatory response. Which one of the following options is the sign of inflammation that is most likely to occur last?
   A Heat
   B Loss of function
   C Pain
   D Redness
   E Swelling

10. During immune responses to invasion of body tissues by micro-organisms, specific antibodies and antitoxins are present and provide immunity against the diseases caused by particular micro-organisms. Which one of the following options is the term used to describe the random inheritance of certain antibodies and antitoxins?
    A Acquired immunity
    B Mutation
    C Natural immunity
    D Passive immunity
    E Vaccination

11. During immune responses to invasion of body tissues by micro-organisms, specific antibodies and antitoxins are present and provide immunity against the diseases caused by particular micro-organisms. Which one of the following options is the term used to describe how a pathogen alters its chemical make-up to produce a new variant of a disease?
    A Acquired immunity
    B Mutation
    C Natural immunity
    D Passive immunity
    E Vaccination

12. The dental team may be exposed to many infections during their normal working lives, due to the close-up and hands-on nature of dentistry. Vaccination against certain diseases is therefore mandatory when working in the clinical environment. Which one of the following options is a vaccination that provides immunity against a pathogen responsible for an infection of the protective tissues surrounding the brain and spinal cord?
    A Hepatitis B
    B Meningitis
    C Mumps
    D Poliomyelitis
    E Tetanus

13. There are many diseases, lesions and conditions that can occur in the oral cavity, some of which are caused by micro-organisms and others that are not. Which one of the following options is a lesion that is not associated with infection by a micro-organism?
    A Apthous ulcer
    B Dental caries
    C Herpetic ulcer
    D Periapical abscess
    E Periodontal abscess

14. Oral cancer is currently one of the few types of cancer whose incidence is increasing in the United Kingdom, and the dental team are in a unique position to identify suspicious lesions at an early stage. Which one of the following options is a known risk factor for oral cancer that is not amenable to lifestyle choice advice by the dental team?
    A Alcohol intake
    B Dietary intake
    C Genetic predisposition
    D Sunlight exposure
    E Tobacco use

15. Various pre-existing medical conditions can have a detrimental effect on the oral soft tissues, either directly or due to drugs involved in their management. Which one of the following options is an oral condition most likely to be seen in a patient with diabetes?
    A Candidiasis
    B Gingival hyperplasia
    C Herpes labialis
    D Poor wound healing
    E Xerostomia

16. Dental caries is a bacterial infection of the mineralised tissues of the tooth which can often result in pain and eventual tooth loss. Which one of the following options is a factor not associated with the onset of dental caries in a tooth?
    A Citric acid
    B Lactic acid
    C Repeated acid exposure
    D Staphylococcal bacteria
    E Sucrose

17. Some foods/drinks can be turned into weak organic acids by oral bacteria and therefore are involved in the process of caries development and cavity formation in teeth. Which one of the following options is a food/drink that is most likely to be involved in the development of dental caries?
    A Semi-skimmed milk
    B Strawberry smoothie

C Sweet potato
D Whole milk
E Whole peach

18. There are many sugar 'alternatives' available in supermarkets and health food shops, some of which are able to cause dental caries. Which one of the following options is an example of an alternative sugar that is not associated with the onset of dental caries?
 A Agave nectar
 B Coconut sugar
 C Honey
 D Milk sugar
 E Syrup

19. Oral bacteria digest the carbohydrate foods that we eat and produce weak organic acids that lower the pH level of the oral cavity such that the tooth structure can be damaged and dental caries can occur. Which one of the following options is the critical pH value at which this acidic damage to the tooth structure begins?
 A pH 5.0
 B pH 5.5
 C pH 6.0
 D pH 6.5
 E pH 7.0

20. Oral bacteria digest the carbohydrate foods that we eat and produce weak organic acids that lower the pH level of the oral cavity such that the tooth structure can be damaged and dental caries can occur. Which one of the following options is the term used to describe the initial damage to the tooth structure that occurs during this process?
 A Cavitation
 B Demineralisation
 C Neutralisation
 D Remineralisation
 E Salivation

21. All food products entering the oral cavity may become stuck in difficult-to-clean points called stagnation areas, therefore increasing the risk of damage to the oral health of the patient. Which one of the following options is a stagnation area that is most likely to be associated with the onset of periodontal disease in the absence of regular and effective cleaning?
 A Buccal pit
 B Crown margin
 C Denture clasp
 D Gingival crevice
 E Occlusal fissure

22. The stages involved in the progression of dental caries within a tooth tend to follow a similar pattern when a previously sound, healthy tooth is attacked. Which one of the following options is the stage most likely to be associated with the onset of hot, cold or sweet sensitivity in the tooth?
    A Alveolar abscess
    B Carious exposure
    C Demineralisation
    D Irreversible pulpitis
    E Reversible pulpitis

23. The enamel surface of teeth can be damaged and lost due to various causes. Which one of the following options is a cause of tooth surface loss often associated with a diet high in acidic foods and drinks?
    A Abfraction
    B Abrasion
    C Attrition
    D Caries
    E Erosion

24. Dental caries is a bacterial infection of the hard tissues of a tooth, while periodontal disease is a bacterial infection of the supporting structures of a tooth. Which one of the following options is a true statement in relation to the onset of both these common oral diseases?
    A Involve anaerobic bacteria only
    B Involve the same species of bacteria
    C Involve thin, watery saliva
    D Occur in the presence of plaque biofilm
    E Occur in the presence of sugars

25. When plaque accumulates around the gingival margins of teeth over a prolonged period without removal, the condition of chronic gingivitis is likely to develop. Which one of the following options is a feature that is not likely to be seen in a patient with chronic gingivitis?
    A Bleeding on probing
    B Gingival inflammation
    C Plaque
    D Swollen papillae
    E True pockets

26. When left untreated, chronic gingivitis will gradually develop into chronic periodontitis, where all of the supporting structures of a tooth will become affected and the tooth may eventually be lost. Which one of the following options is an event that is most likely to also occur in the absence of chronic periodontitis?
    A Formation of true pocket
    B Gingival recession

C Loss of soft tissue attachment
D Tooth mobility
E Toxin passage through micro-ulcers

27. Periodontal disease is one of the most common diseases throughout civilisation, and there are various known contributory factors to its level of severity, when present. Which one of the following options is the factor that is the actual cause of periodontal disease, rather than a contributory factor to the severity of the disease?
A Hormonal imbalance
B Immunocompromised
C Mouth breathing
D Poor oral hygiene
E Smoking

Extended matching questions

For each of the following dental pathology and microbiology questions, select the single most appropriate answer from the option list. Each option might be used once, more than once or not at all.

a) Actinomyces species
b) Alveolar abscess
c) Apthous ulcer
d) Candida albicans
e) Cellulitis
f) Dentigerous cyst
g) Legionella
h) Lichen planus
i) Periodontitis
j) Squamous cell carcinoma
k) *Streptococcus mutans*

1. Radiographs are useful diagnostic aids for the dental team, as they allow oral areas and structures to be visualised that are normally not visible. Unseen lesions can then be seen and treated successfully by the dental team. Which one of the options listed is the most likely lesion to be present when a periapical radiograph reveals a black, circular area around the root apex of an upper incisor tooth?

2. A patient has failed to attend for several appointments to have a grossly carious lower molar tooth surgically extracted, and he is now suffering from a second episode of intense pain and swelling around the tooth. On examination the dentist realises that the swelling is extending beyond the local area of the tooth, and the patient admits he is having difficulty in swallowing. Which one of the options listed is the most likely condition to be present in this scenario?

3. Ulceration may occur anywhere in the digestive system, from the mouth to the large intestines, and lesions may also occur on the skin. Which one of the options listed is the term used to describe the specific oral lesions associated with an ulcerative disorder of the skin where the oral lesions are recognised as being pre-malignant?

4. Dental caries is a bacterial infection of the hard tissues of the teeth, and its rampant occurrence and treatment by tooth extraction in younger patients accounts for the majority of general anaesthetic admissions of children in the United Kingdom. Which one of the options listed is the most prevalent micro-organism associated with an initial carious lesion in a tooth?

Answers

Multiple choice questions

1. *The correct answer is A.* Each bacterium exists as an organism made up of just one cell, with a rigid outer wall that determines its shape and helps to categorise similar-shaped bacteria into named groups.

2. *The correct answer is C.* This group of chemicals acts specifically against bacteria (rather than fungi or viruses) and kills the micro-organisms rather than just preventing their spread by reproduction.

3. *The correct answer is D.* This virus has recently been linked to some cases of oral cancer, particularly those occurring in the oropharyngeal area of the mouth. The British Dental Association joined other organisations to successfully campaign for the widespread and ongoing immunisation of all teenage boys and girls against the virus in the UK.

4. *The correct answer is C.* Many people develop immunity from the virus after suffering a bout of chickenpox as a child, but not all do so, and a vaccine is now available as the disease tends to be more serious in adults.

5. *The correct answer is C.* This is the only fungal infection of any importance to affect the oral soft tissues, causing several lesions and diseases including oral thrush and angular cheilitis.

6. *The correct answer is D.* The swelling produced may cause no harm to the surrounding tissues and be classed as a benign tumour, or it may allow invasion and damage to the surrounding tissues and be classed as a malignant tumour.

7. *The correct answer is C.* Early carious lesions are usually associated with bacterial infection by *Streptococcus mutans*, and then other micro-organisms such as *Lactobacilli* are present as the cavity deepens.

8. *The correct answer is D.* The inability to remove the white patch from the mucosa by wiping excludes a diagnosis of an infection with *Candida* and makes the presence of the white patch a potentially more serious condition, as leukoplakias are regarded as potentially pre-malignant. However, they sometimes have no sinister consequences and very often no obvious cause either.

9. *The correct answer is B.* On exposure to an irritant, the body reacts by increasing the blood flow to the area – this results in the area becoming red, warm to touch and swollen. The swelling presses on the surrounding nerves, causing pain, and when the pain becomes too intense, there is a loss of function of the tissue.

10. *The correct answer is C.* Natural immunity is present from birth and is completely randomly inherited. Individuals so affected are able to survive certain diseases that others cannot, hence providing a natural pool of antibodies and antitoxins that can be developed into vaccines for administration to the general population.

11. *The correct answer is B.* Viruses are especially difficult to treat with vaccinations as they mutate so readily. During the coronavirus pandemic of 2020–2021, several mutations occurred during the UK's mass vaccination programme and produced variants of the virus – the South African variant, the Brazilian variant and the Indian variant to name but a few.

12. *The correct answer is B.* Childhood vaccination against meningitis is now routine in the UK.

13. *The correct answer is A.* Apthous ulcers are shallow breaks in the mucous membrane of the oral cavity and are not associated with an infection. They are very painful, and sufferers often have recurrent attacks. The ulcers may be small (minor) or larger (major) and have been linked to stress and nutritional deficiencies in some patients.

14. *The correct answer is C.* Some patients are unfortunate enough to have a genetic predisposition for developing some types of cancer – some defect or alteration of their genes makes them more likely to develop certain cancers than the average person. While all other options may be discussed and advice and recommendations given by the team to make healthier lifestyle choices, nothing can alter the patient's genetic make-up.

15. *The correct answer is D.* Diabetic patients suffer from a reduced peripheral blood flow as part of the disease, so the oral cavity and the skin of the hands, legs and feet have a reduced supply of oxygenated blood. Following injury or when an infection is present, this blood flow reduction affects the patient's ability to heal fully, and diabetics often suffer from prolonged healing after treatment such as an extraction.

16. *The correct answer is D.* Staphylococcal bacteria are associated with skin and mucous membrane lesions, such as boils and impetigo. Streptococcal bacteria are associated with early carious lesions.

17. *The correct answer is B.* When fresh fruits are blended to make a smoothie, the cell wall structure of the natural fruit is destroyed and the carbohydrate content is released as free sugars. While less cariogenic than foods and drinks such as cakes and fizzy pop, smoothies should be confined to mealtimes only and followed by brushing or mouth washing. Juiced fresh fruits pose a similar risk of causing dental caries.

18. *The correct answer is D.* Milk sugar, or lactose, is non-cariogenic when taken in an unsweetened form. All other options are cariogenic alternatives to sugar.

19. *The correct answer is B.* pH 5.5 is actually referred to as the 'critical pH' by the dental team.

20. *The correct answer is B.* The weak organic acids remove the crystalline mineral content of the enamel prisms so that the enamel surface becomes demineralised. Neutralisation of the acids occurs when the pH level returns to 7, and

then remineralisation can occur, where the damage to the enamel structure is repaired. If demineralisation occurs more frequently than remineralisation a cavity will eventually form.

21. *The correct answer is D.* Periodontal disease affects the supporting structures of the teeth, including the gingivae. The gingival crevice acts as a stagnation area for food debris and then plaque, resulting in gingivitis and then periodontitis. All other options are stagnation areas affecting the tooth itself and will result in caries.

22. *The correct answer is E.* The caries is within the dentine layer of the tooth, and the nerve fibrils in this structure will respond to thermal and sweet stimulation. If the caries is treated at this point by removal and tooth restoration, the tooth should settle and become fully functional again.

23. *The correct answer is E.* Erosion is one of the non-carious tooth surface loss factors that can cause tooth damage and is due to the action of extrinsic (dietary) acid on the enamel. Extrinsic acids are those ingested by the patient rather than the intrinsic acids produced by oral bacteria during food and drink intake.

24. *The correct answer is D.* When a plaque biofilm builds on a tooth surface and is not removed, caries develops. When the biofilm develops in the gingival crevice and subgingivally, periodontal disease develops. Sugars are necessary for the onset of caries only, and the bacteria involved in both diseases are different.

25. *The correct answer is E.* True pockets are present when the periodontal ligament is destroyed and the tooth has lost its attachment to the supporting structures – this is a feature of periodontitis, not gingivitis.

26. *The correct answer is B.* Gingival recession can also occur as a natural ageing process without chronic periodontitis being present and as a result of excessive toothbrushing such as occurs in patients with abrasion damage to their teeth. Again, chronic periodontitis is often not present in these patients.

27. *The correct answer is D.* The accumulation of bacterial plaque due to poor oral hygiene is the causative factor of periodontal disease. All other options are contributory factors to the level of its severity when already present.

Extended matching questions

1. *The correct answer is b).* An alveolar abscess occurs when the pulp of a tooth dies and the resulting dead tissue, infective material and pus pass out of the apical foramen of the tooth and collect around the root apex. Its radiographic appearance is usually diagnostic, and the treatment options for the tooth will either be pulpectomy and restoration or extraction.

2. *The correct answer is e).* Untreated dental disease and abscesses have the potential to spread into the surrounding soft tissue areas and cause serious complications for the patient. Although antibiotics may alleviate the symptoms of the infection for a time, dental treatment must always be carried out to treat or remove the source of the infection as soon as possible to prevent such serious complications.

3. *The correct answer is h).* Oral lesions are relatively common with lichen planus, and they classically appear as lacy white striae on the buccal mucosa, although sometimes they may become ulcerative. Biopsy will confirm the diagnosis.

4. *The correct answer is k).* Research has shown that *Streptococcus mutans* is the bacterium usually associated with an early carious lesion in any tooth and wherever the lesion first forms. It is also the micro-organism responsible for the production of the majority of the weak organic acids that cause enamel demineralisation.

9a Assessment and Diagnosis

Multiple choice questions

1. Oral health assessments are carried out each time that a patient attends the dental practice but particularly when patients attend for an examination. Various templates for recording assessment findings may be used by the team, and all should broadly cover the areas listed below. Which one of the following options is the most likely area where pocket depths are recorded?
   A Dentition
   B Extra-oral tissues
   C Intra-oral tissues
   D Occlusion
   E Periodontal tissues

2. Oral health assessments are carried out each time that a patient attends the dental practice but particularly when patients attend for an examination. Various templates for recording assessment findings may be used by the team, and all should broadly cover the areas listed below. Which one of the following options is the most likely area where the presence of a suspected squamous cell carcinoma lesion is recorded?
   A Dentition
   B Extra-oral tissues
   C Intra-oral tissues
   D Occlusion
   E Periodontal tissues

3. There are many methods available to the dental team for carrying out a particular aspect of an oral health assessment, ranging from basic vision to the use of radiographs. Which one of the following options is an assessment method most likely to be used to assess the occlusal classification of a patient?
   A BPE probe
   B Briault probe

Questions and Answers for Dental Nurses, Fourth Edition. Carole Hollins.

C Intra-oral photograph
D Study models
E Transillumination

4. There are many methods available to the dental team for carrying out a particular aspect of an oral health assessment, ranging from basic vision to the use of radiographs. Which one of the following options is an assessment method most likely to be used to detect a lateral periodontal abscess?
   A Dental panoramic tomograph
   B Intra-oral photograph
   C Periapical radiograph
   D Study models
   E Vitality test

5. There are many hand instruments used by dental professionals while carrying out an oral health assessment, including mouth mirrors and various probes. Which one of the following options is not a recognised use of a mouth mirror?
   A Detecting soft dentine
   B Protecting soft tissues
   C Providing vision
   D Reflecting light
   E Retracting soft tissues

6. One area considered during an oral health assessment is the occlusion of the patient's teeth: the way the teeth bite together and whether this is normal or whether a malocclusion is present. Which one of the following options is the term used during this assessment to describe a malocclusion where the lower jaw is further forward than normal?
   A Class I
   B Class II
   C Class II division 1
   D Class II division 2
   E Class III

7. One area considered during an oral health assessment is the occlusion of the patient's teeth: the way the teeth bite together and whether this is normal or whether a malocclusion is present. Which one of the following options is the term used during this assessment to describe the vertical overlap of the lower incisors by the upper incisors?
   A Angle's classification
   B Crowding
   C Malocclusion
   D Overbite
   E Overjet

8. The periodontal tissues are those acting as the supporting structures of the teeth, and they are routinely assessed for signs of disease during an oral health assessment. Which one of the following options is a hand instrument not used during a periodontal assessment of a patient?
   A BPE probe
   B Briault probe
   C CPITN probe
   D UNC probe
   E WHO probe

9. The periodontal tissues are those acting as the supporting structures of the teeth, and they are routinely assessed for signs of disease during an oral health assessment. A basic periodontal examination (BPE) is carried out initially to identify areas requiring further periodontal investigation. Which one of the following options is the BPE code that indicates the presence of plaque retention factors?
   A Code 0
   B Code 1
   C Code 2
   D Code 3
   E Code 4

10. Dental radiography is an important diagnostic tool used during oral health assessments to help diagnose the cause of dental problems and to help avoid problems during dental treatment. Which one of the following options is a radiograph view most likely to be used to detect the presence and position of a 'mesiodens' supernumerary tooth?
    A Anterior occlusal
    B Horizontal bitewing
    C Lateral oblique
    D Periapical (child size)
    E Vertical bitewing

11. Dental radiography is an important diagnostic tool used during oral health assessments to help diagnose the cause of dental problems and to help avoid problems during dental treatment. Which one of the following options is the radiograph view most likely to be used to check for the presence of restoration overhangs of the left posterior sextants?
    A Anterior occlusal
    B Horizontal bitewing
    C Lateral oblique
    D Periapical
    E Vertical bitewing

12. Dental radiography is an important diagnostic tool used during oral health assessments and can be carried out using both conventional and digital techniques.

Which one of the following options is an advantage of a conventional radiograph over a digital one?

A Image can be shared electronically
B Image can be stored as hard copy
C Image cannot be altered
D Lower radiation dose
E No chemicals are required

13. An X-ray film packet is made up of various components, each with their own role to play in the correct formation of an image when the packet is exposed to X-radiation. Which one of the following options is the most likely component that is present to absorb scattered radiation during exposure?

A Black paper
B Celluloid sheet
C Lead foil
D Plastic envelope
E Silver bromide

14. Non-digital radiographs must be mounted correctly for viewing, otherwise incorrect tooth identification and treatment may occur. Location markers are used to help achieve correct mounting, either as raised pimples on intra-oral films or the letters 'R' or 'L' on extra-oral films. Which one of the following options describes the correct mounting for a periapical view of the upper left incisors?

A Pimple in, roots above crowns, central incisor towards centreline
B Pimple in, roots below crowns, lateral incisor towards centreline
C Pimple out, roots above crowns, central incisor away from centreline
D Pimple out, roots above crowns, lateral incisor away from centreline
E Pimple out, roots below crowns, lateral incisor away from centreline

15. Non-digital radiographs may undergo various errors during exposure, handling and processing, many of which render them unreadable by the clinician. Which one of the following options is an exposure fault due to the collimator being positioned at too shallow an angle to the film packet?

A Blurring
B Coning
C Elongation
D Fogging
E Foreshortening

16. An X-ray film packet is made up of various components, each with their own role to play in the correct formation of an image when the packet is exposed to X-radiation. Which one of the following options is the most likely component that is present to allow the image to be stored permanently, once processed?

A Black paper
B Celluloid sheet
C Lead foil
D Plastic envelope
E Silver bromide

Extended matching questions

For each of the following oral health assessment and diagnosis questions, select the single most appropriate answer from the option list. Each option might be used once, more than once or not at all.

a) 17
b) 42
c) 55
d) Class II division 1
e) Class II division 2
f) Class III
g) Code 2
h) Code 3
i) Code 4
j) Complete overbite
k) LL5
l) Posterior crossbite
m) Reverse overjet
n) UL7
o) UR5

1. A teenager has undergone an orthodontic assessment with the dentist as he dislikes the appearance of his teeth and would like them straightened. In particular, the patient complains that when he bites together his upper front teeth are behind his lowers. Which one of the options listed is the most likely malocclusion to be present in this case?

2. During an oral health assessment, the patient's periodontal tissues are examined and a record made of any findings. Which one of the options listed is the most likely BPE notation to be used when a pocket up to 5.5 mm deep has been found during the examination?

3. A new dentist has started working at the practice after graduating in North America the previous year. On completing a dental examination on a patient, the dentist has found a cavity and records it as a mesio-occlusal in tooth 15 using the Universal charting system. Which one of the options listed is the most likely charting for this tooth using the alphanumeric system?

4. After carrying out an orthodontic assessment of a teenage patient, the dentist has noted that the lower first molars and canine teeth are behind their normal occlusal positions and the patient has an overjet of 9 mm. Which one of the options listed is the most likely malocclusion to be present in this patient?

5. A young boy has undergone a dental examination and the dentist has discovered a small cavity developing in the child's upper right second deciduous molar tooth. Which one of the options listed is the most likely charting notation of this tooth in the FDI system?

Answers

Multiple choice questions

1. *The correct answer is E.* True pockets are likely to be present when a patient has periodontal disease – a bacterial infection of the supporting structures of the teeth. The depth and location of the pockets are recorded to determine the severity of the disease and guide the dentist towards a treatment plan.

2. *The correct answer is C.* These lesions are the most common oral cancers seen, and they affect the oral soft tissues, particularly the tongue borders and the floor of the mouth, although they can occur elsewhere in the mouth. Soft tissue 'mouth maps' are often used to record the exact site of any lesion, and many dentists also use intra-oral photography to provide specialists with an image for referral purposes too.

3. *The correct answer is D.* Study models are a set of stone casts made from upper and lower impressions taken of the patient's teeth that, together with a bite recording, can be held in the occlusal position of the jaws of that patient by the dentist. The occlusion and individual tooth positions can then be viewed from all angles, including from the back of the models (which is an impossible angle to view within the patient's mouth) so that the occlusal classification can be determined.

4. *The correct answer is C.* This radiographic view shows one or two teeth in full length, from the crown top to the root apex and the surrounding bone. A lateral periodontal abscess will be visible as a darkened area at the base of a periodontal pocket on the side of the root of the tooth. An alveolar abscess will be visible as a circular darkened area at the root apex.

5. *The correct answer is A.* A tooth probe is required to detect soft dentine, by being scratched over the dentine surface so that hard dentine will make a 'scratchy' noise while soft dentine will not.

6. *The correct answer is E.* This is a discrepancy of the jaw relationship, where the forward position of the lower jaw often results in a reverse overjet – the lower anterior teeth close in front of the upper anterior teeth, and the patient often has a prominent chin. In milder cases the anterior teeth may bite edge to edge.

7. *The correct answer is D.* The overbite is measured as the vertical amount of coverage of the lower central incisors by the upper central incisors, as a percentage. An average overbite is 50%, a higher percentage indicates more of the lower teeth are covered by the uppers than normal, while a lower percentage indicates less coverage up to 0%, where the patient bites in an edge-to-edge position.

8. *The correct answer is B.* A Briault probe is a double-ended probe used to detect cavities or soft dentine lying in the mesial or distal surfaces of the teeth, especially the posterior teeth. All other options are types of periodontal probes.

9. *The correct answer is C.* Code 2 indicates that either supragingival or subgingival calculus is present, or some other plaque retention factor such as an overhanging restoration. Any pockets present are no more than 3.5 mm deep.

10. *The correct answer is A.* The view can be taken using an anterior occlusal film or an adult-size periapical film. The film is placed horizontally between the anterior upper and lower teeth and exposed in a direction roughly perpendicular to the bridge of the nose so that the upper teeth are seen in full length on the film. The mesiodens will appear between the roots of the upper central incisors if one is present.

11. *The correct answer is B.* The horizontal bitewing will show an image of the crowns of the upper and lower posterior teeth and their bony interdental crests on one radiograph. Any restorations extending into the interdental areas, where overhangs are most likely to occur, will therefore be visible.

12. *The correct answer is C.* Digital images are transmitted to a computer for viewing rather than being processed as a hard copy radiograph, as for a conventional image. However, various computer software programmes allow alteration of the digital image in the same way that digital photographs can be altered and enhanced. This may cause problems in dentolegal litigation cases as treatment results can be enhanced or altered.

13. *The correct answer is C.* Lead is a metallic chemical element that is dense enough to prevent the passage of X-radiation through it. It is present as a thin, flexible foil within the film packet, on the side of the celluloid film away from the direction of the X-ray exposure. Any X-rays not absorbed by the tissues being exposed are absorbed by the lead foil rather than being allowed to scatter into the surrounding area.

14. *The correct answer is D.* The pimple must always be out, towards the person viewing the radiograph. The central incisor is always towards the centreline, and for upper incisors the roots should be above the crowns of the teeth.

15. *The correct answer is C.* When the collimator angle is too shallow, the X-rays can be visualised as skimming along the surface of the film and producing an overly long image, in the same way as the sun lying low in the sky at dusk produces an elongated shadow of a tree, or a person or building, for example.

16. *The correct answer is B.* The celluloid film is coated with light-sensitive silver bromide salts in an emulsion that produce the latent image on the film when exposed to X-rays. The processing chemicals then react with the salts to produce the permanent image on the film.

Extended matching questions

1. *The correct answer is f).* A reverse overjet, as described, occurs in class III malocclusions where the mandible is further forward of its normal position.

2. *The correct answer is h).* Code 2 records pockets up to 3.5 mm and the presence of plaque retention factors, while code 4 records pockets greater than 5.5 mm.

3. *The correct answer is n).* The Universal charting system charts the teeth from 1 to 32, starting on the upper right, then upper left, then lower left to lower right. So UR8 is '1', UL8 is '16', LL8 is '17' and LR8 is '32'. Tooth '15' then is UL7.

4. *The correct answer is d).* Class II division 1 malocclusions occur when the mandible occludes too far back from the normal class I position so that the lower lip lies behind the upper incisor teeth. This allows these teeth to splay forward so that the overjet is greater than 4 mm. In severe cases the overjet can be measured into the teens of millimetres.

5. *The correct answer is c).* The FDI charting system scores teeth in a two-digit method from the upper right clockwise to the lower right – the first digit being the quadrant and the second being the tooth number. In adults then, the upper right quadrant is 1, upper left is 2, lower left is 3 and lower right is 4. When deciduous teeth are present the upper right quadrant is 5, the upper left is 6, the lower left is 7 and the lower right is 8. The second deciduous molar is the fifth tooth posteriorly from the midline, so on the upper right it is charted as 55.

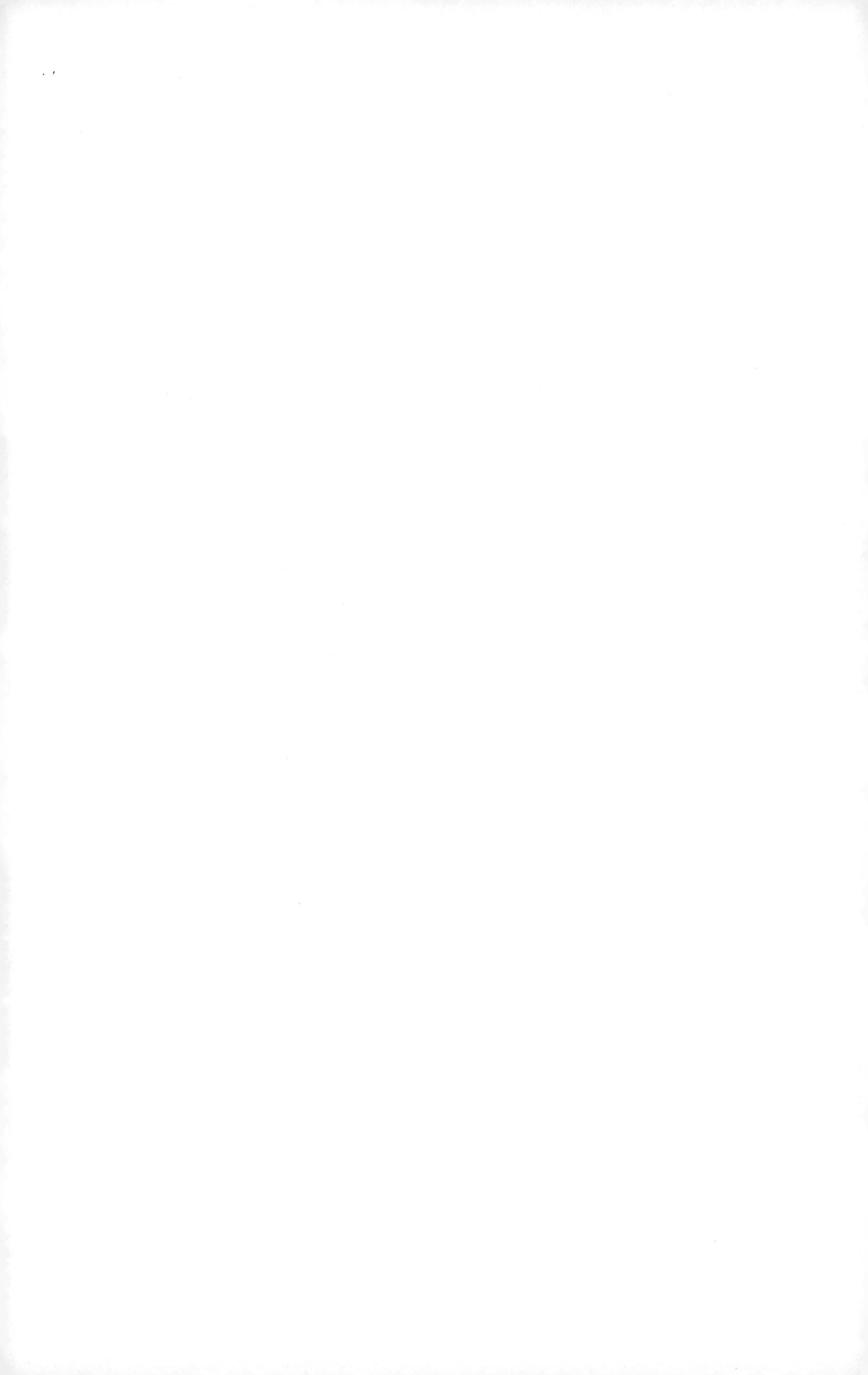

10 Restorative Dentistry and Dental Materials

Multiple choice questions

1. When a tooth undergoes a carious attack, a cavity is formed, and these are classified into five different types, dependent on the site of the original caries. Which one of the following options is an example of a class III cavity in a tooth?
   - A Buccal pit of molar
   - B Cervical margin of premolar
   - C Distal surface of canine
   - D Labial surface of incisor
   - E Mesio-occlusal surfaces of molar

2. Permanent filling materials are used to restore teeth to their appearance and full function after a cavity has been cleared of caries and prepared to receive the filling, while temporary filling materials are used to seal a cavity for a time. The materials available are either plastic or pre-constructed. Which one of the following options is an example of a pre-constructed filling material?
   - A Amalgam
   - B Composite
   - C Glass ionomer
   - D Porcelain
   - E Zinc oxide/eugenol

3. Providing adequate moisture control during restorative procedures is one of the most important duties of the dental nurse and enables the operator to restore teeth safely and effectively. Which one of the following options is the moisture control technique most effective at removing aerosols from the operative field during a restorative procedure?
   - A Absorbent material use
   - B Compressed air drying
   - C High-volume aspiration

Questions and Answers for Dental Nurses, Fourth Edition. Carole Hollins.

D Low-volume aspiration
E Rubber dam

4. Rubber dam is a method of moisture control used widely in dentistry, particularly for endodontic procedures. Its use isolates the tooth under treatment from the rest of the oral cavity and protects the patient's airway from fluids, debris and instruments. Which one of the following options is the rubber dam kit instrument used to pierce the hole so that a tooth can be isolated for treatment?
   A Dam clamp
   B Dam forceps
   C Dam frame
   D Dam punch
   E Dam sheet

5. Composite filling materials are tooth-coloured restoratives that are available in a wide range of shades, enabling them to be matched to a patient's tooth colour when used. The majority are light-cured and contain an inorganic filler, resin and a catalyst that is activated when exposed to the curing light at the chairside. Which one of the following options is an example of a composite material used to allow superior polishing and a gloss finish in anterior teeth?
   A Bulk-fill composite
   B Hybrid composite
   C Microfine composite
   D Nano composite
   E Universal composite

6. Glass ionomer filling materials are tooth-coloured restoratives that are adhesive to all the hard tissues of the teeth and so tend to be used in situations where little natural retention of a restoration is available. Which one of the following options is an example of a particular use of a glass ionomer restoration due to its adhesive properties?
   A Class I cavity
   B Class II cavity
   C Class III cavity
   D Class IV cavity
   E Class V cavity

7. Endodontics is the term used in dentistry for procedures carried out inside a tooth involving treatment to, or the partial or full removal of, the pulp tissue. Endodontic procedures may be non-surgical or surgical. Which one of the following options is an endodontic procedure that involves the placing of a retrograde root filling?
   A Apicectomy
   B Pulp capping
   C Pulpectomy

D Pulpotomy
E Root canal therapy

8. There are many instruments, items and materials used in endodontics that have specific uses during the course of a root canal therapy procedure. Which one of the following options is a material used to obturate the pulp canal?
   A Antiseptic paste
   B Calcium hydroxide
   C Calcium silicate
   D Gutta percha
   E Paper

9. Occasionally a carious cavity extends deep into a tooth and results in an exposure of the pulp chamber. If the exposure is small the dentist may decide to cover the area with a biocompatible material such as calcium silicate, before temporising the tooth for a time. Which one of the following options is the most likely purpose of placing the biocompatible material in this situation?
   A Allow dentine repair
   B Allow future restoration
   C Avoid extraction
   D Disinfect pulp tissue
   E Kill pulp tissue

10. After a permanent filling has been placed in a tooth the operator should check the patient's occlusion to ensure that the new restoration is not preventing them from closing their teeth together fully. When a problem is found in this situation it is referred to as a premature contact. Which one of the following options is an item that is used to identify a premature contact on a new filling?
   A Acetate strip
   B Articulating paper
   C Finishing strip
   D Gutta percha point
   E Wooden wedge

11. Composite materials have been widely available in dentistry for many years and are likely to be used as restoratives more frequently still, as amalgam is gradually phased out of use. They are also available in a range of shades so that the operator can match a restorative to the patient's tooth colour at each use. Which one of the following options is a constituent found in all composite materials, irrespective of its reason for use or its shade?
   A Calcium hydroxide
   B Inorganic filler
   C Quartz and polyacrylate
   D Resin and silver
   E Silver and quartz

12. When a class II cavity is being restored in a tooth, the operator must ensure that no filling material becomes lodged accidentally in the interdental area as once set, it may act as a plaque retention factor and cause periodontal problems in future. Which one of the following options is an item that can be used to prevent this from happening while the restoration is being placed?
    - A Articulating paper
    - B Finishing strip
    - C Matrix outfit
    - D Retraction cord
    - E Rubber dam

13. When a composite restoration is placed in a tooth, the enamel requires etching first to chemically roughen its surface and ensure a good bond is created between the filling material and the tooth structure. Which one of the following options is the material used to etch the enamel in this situation?
    - A Hydrochloric acid
    - B Hydrogen peroxide
    - C Phosphoric acid
    - D Polyacrylic acid
    - E Sodium hypochlorite

14. When a patient presents for treatment of a deep cavity in a tooth, the operator must attempt to remove as much of the carious dentine as possible without breaching the pulp chamber and causing an exposure. Which one of the following items is most likely to be used to remove the deepest areas of carious dentine from a cavity?
    - A Ball-ended burnisher
    - B Diamond fissure bur
    - C Flat plastic
    - D Spoon excavator
    - E Stainless steel rose-head bur

15. Most operators have a selection of hand instruments laid out on a conservation tray while performing restorative treatments, and each instrument has a specific purpose during the procedure. Some instruments are always used while others are only used for certain materials. Which one of the following options is an instrument that can be used for soft tissue retraction and to improve visibility in the operative area?
    - A Ball-ended burnisher
    - B Flat plastic
    - C Large excavator
    - D Mouth mirror
    - E Plugger

Extended matching questions

Topic: I

For each of the following restorative dentistry and dental materials questions, select the requested number of most appropriate answers from the option list. Each option might be used once, more than once or not at all.

a) Acetate strip
b) Cermet
c) Cervical acetate matrix
d) Cervical foil matrix
e) Finishing strip
f) Flowable composite
g) Friction grip finishing bur
h) Friction grip fissure bur
i) Hybrid composite
j) Latch grip polishing disc
k) Latch grip rose-head bur
l) Resin bond
m) Resin-modified glass ionomer

1. A patient has attended for a class III composite restoration to be replaced in her upper left central incisor, as the current restoration is discoloured and looks unsightly. Which one of the options listed is the most likely item to be used to ensure that the new restoration is adapted correctly to the tooth in the interdental area?

2. A child of 8 years has attended for his first dental examination at the practice, and the dentist is pleased to see that he has no cavities, good oral hygiene and is at the correct stage of mixed dentition for his age. The dentist advises that all four of the child's permanent first molar teeth be fissure sealed as a preventative measure against future caries, and he and his mother agree. Which three of the options listed are the most likely examples of suitable restorative materials that can be used for this purpose?

3. A patient is undergoing a restorative procedure on the upper right first premolar tooth, which is previously restored and has recurrent caries present. Once the old filling and the caries have been removed, just the palatal wall of the tooth remains, and the dentist and patient decide that the tooth now needs to have a core rebuild and then a crown placed in the near future. Which two of the options listed are suitable materials to be used for the core rebuild procedure?

Topic: II

For each of the following restorative dentistry and dental materials questions, select the requested number of most appropriate answers from the option list. Each option might be used once, more than once or not at all.

a) Apex locater
b) Engine file
c) Finger spreader
d) Gates Glidden drill
e) Gutta percha point
f) Paper point
g) Pulp capping
h) Pulpectomy
i) Pulpotomy
j) Rotary paste filler
k) Ruler

1. The dentist has successfully cleaned, shaped and prepared a patient's upper canine tooth during a pulpectomy procedure and is now ready to place the root filling. Which three of the options listed are the most likely items that will be required to dry the canal, then apply a sealant material and then obturate the canal?

2. A patient attends the practice with a fractured upper premolar tooth requesting that the dentist tries to save it if possible. The patient has no pain, and a periapical radiograph reveals that the tooth has been successfully root filled previously, so the dentist suggests placing a pre-formed post into the tooth and then rebuilding it. Which one of the options listed is the most likely item to be used to remove some existing gutta percha material and make room for the new post?

3. A dentist is carrying out a root canal procedure on a patient who attended previously with the symptoms of irreversible pulpitis. The tooth was opened and debrided, then dressed with an antiseptic paste for several weeks while the patient went on holiday. As the tooth has settled fully it is now being root filled. Which three of the options listed are the most likely items that can be used to determine the working length of the root canal?

Answers

Multiple choice questions

1. *The correct answer is C.* Class III cavities involve the mesial or distal surface of any anterior teeth, that is, the incisors and canines.

2. *The correct answer is D.* The word 'plastic' in this context indicates the materials are malleable – they are not solid and can be manipulated into shape before setting. This applies to all the options listed except porcelain, which is a material used in the laboratory to form a pre-constructed filling from a prepared study model cast of the cavity.

3. *The correct answer is C.* High-volume aspiration actively sucks aerosols away from the operative field and into the suction system within the surgery. Rubber dam does not remove aerosols from the area but does limit the contamination of the area by the patient's breath during treatment.

4. *The correct answer is D.* The dam punch has a rotary disc of graded holes that is used to select the size of hole required (from small incisor to large molar). The dam material is placed across the disc in a single sheet, and the handles are squeezed together to activate the punch head, which cuts a hole through the dam sheet.

5. *The correct answer is C.* The inorganic filler consists of very small-sized, round particles that allow a superior polish compared to other composites and results in a gloss finish that mimics shiny enamel.

6. *The correct answer is E.* Class V cavities are those present at the cervical margin of any tooth, where there is little enamel present. Glass ionomers are adhesive to all hard tissues of the teeth so provide maximum retention in this situation, compared to composites.

7. *The correct answer is A.* This is a surgical endodontic procedure where an apical infection is present but cannot be accessed as normal through the crown of the root. Instead, a surgical flap is raised over the apex of the tooth, and the infectious material and any attached pathology such as a cyst is removed through the bone. The apical end of the root is then root filled – this is the retrograde root filling.

8. *The correct answer is D.* Gutta percha is a biologically stable, rubbery material that is radiopaque on radiographs. It is available as various length and width tapered cones that match the length and width of endodontic files and reamers, so that a root canal can be filled (obturated) with a cone matching the file size of the working length of the root.

9. *The correct answer is A.* Biocompatible materials such as calcium silicate promote the formation of a dentine bridge over the pulp chamber when placed into the base of a cavity, by stimulating the odontoblast cells to form secondary dentine. Calcium hydroxide as a liner in deep cavities had a similar function, but research shows the new products are more successful.

10. *The correct answer is B.* Articulating paper is presented as thin strips impregnated with blue or red dye on either side that leave a mark on the tooth at the site of the premature contact. The strip is placed between the teeth and the patient is asked to bite into their normal closed position and then move their jaw from side to side. When coloured marks are left on all of the teeth rather than just the new restoration, the bite is correct.

11. *The correct answer is B.* The inorganic filler is present as a strengthener and may consist of powdered glass, quartz, silica or other ceramic particles but is always present in composite materials.

12. *The correct answer is C.* Matrix outfits, such as Siqveland or Tofflemire, are presented as bands of metal that are inserted around the tooth and tightened against its sides so that no gaps are present between the band and the tooth interdentally. The filling material (usually amalgam with these outfits) can then be inserted into the cavity and manipulated into shape without any spillage into this area. Various similar matrix outfits are also available with bands of acetate for use with posterior composite materials.

13. *The correct answer is C.* A 33% concentration of phosphoric acid is the typical strength of acid etchant products and is available as gels and liquids. They are usually strongly coloured to enable their accurate placement on the tooth or in a cavity only, as the material will cause a chemical burn if it inadvertently contacts soft tissues.

14. *The correct answer is D.* The vast majority of the tooth tissue will be removed by high-speed then low-speed burs, but as the cavity deepens and the pulp chamber is approached, the dentist will resort to the use of hand instruments to continue caries removal. These allow tactile sensation during use, so the dentist can feel when the dentine is hard or soft and can proceed to carefully remove the deeper caries. The spoon excavator instrument was designed for this task.

15. *The correct answer is D.* The soft tissues of the lips, cheeks and the tongue require retraction during a restorative procedure to allow access and good vision and to prevent their injury while drilling is being carried out. A mouth mirror is slimmer than the operator's fingers when retracting soft tissues, and if angled correctly, the mirror can be used to reflect light into the operative field to allow better vision.

Extended matching questions

Topic: I

1. *The correct answer is a).* Acetate strips are available as pre-cut segments or as a full roll that can be cut to a length of choice. Their thin nature and pliability allow them to be easily manipulated into tight interdental areas so that

adjacent teeth are separated from each other and the strip can be folded around the tooth as necessary. As they are clear, the curing light beam passes through the strip during use and cures the restoration beneath.

2. *The correct answers are f), l) and m).* Flowable composites have a reduced inorganic filler content compared to conventional composites so are quite runny before setting, while resin bond is unfilled and very runny. The slight opacity of the flowable composites makes them easier to see and place accurately than the unfilled resins. Resin-modified glass ionomer materials are also easily manipulated into fissures before curing. All three materials can be used for fissure sealing permanent teeth.

3. *The correct answers are b) and i).* Cermets are glass ionomer materials that have been reinforced by the addition of a metal and are for use as core build-up products. The glass ionomer component allows adhesion of the material to both enamel and dentine. Hybrid composites are also suitable for use as core rebuilds, as they have various-sized filler particles to provide greater strength than universal or microfine composite materials.

Topic: II

1. *The correct answers are e), f) and j).* The paper point will be used to dry any residual irrigant solution from the canal before the rotary paste filler is used to spin the sealant material into the canal and smear it on the canal walls. Finally, the correctly sized gutta percha point is inserted to the correct working length within the canal during the obturation stage of the procedure.

2. *The correct answer is d).* Gates Glidden drills are boring instruments, used to bore into root canals and their contents and drill them out, leaving a space available to place pre-formed posts for rebuilds or to have impressions taken for a cast post and core to be constructed.

3. *The correct answers are a), b) and k).* An apex locater is an electronic handpiece that automatically counts down the distance of the engine file tip from the tooth apex, giving the distance in mm. The length of the engine file is known from its gradation marks along the shaft. Alternatively, the working length can be determined manually by taking a paralleled radiograph of the tooth with the pre-measured file in place (using the ruler) and assessing the working length from the image produced.

10a Prosthodontics

Multiple choice questions

1. Alginate impression material is an irreversible hydrocolloid that is elastic in nature, so that it can be used to record areas of undercut in the oral cavity. After an alginate impression has been taken it must be handled and packaged correctly, ready to be sent to the laboratory. Which one of the following options is not a necessary action to take when handling and packaging an alginate impression?
   A Blown dry after disinfection
   B Disinfected by immersion
   C Kept moist for transport
   D Rinsed to remove gross debris
   E Sealed in an airtight bag for transport

2. Prosthodontics is the branch of dentistry concerned with the restoration or replacement of damaged or missing teeth using artificially constructed devices, such as crowns and inlays or dentures and bridges, respectively. In each situation, impressions are taken of the prepared teeth or the dental arches using various impression materials. Which one of the following options is an impression material that is not suitable for use when recording an inlay preparation in a tooth?
   A Addition silicone
   B Alginate
   C Condensation silicone
   D Polyether
   E Vinyl polysiloxane

Questions and Answers for Dental Nurses, Fourth Edition. Carole Hollins.

3. When a tooth is being prepared for a crown, the dentist usually uses a friction grip tapered diamond bur to remove adequate tooth substance for the placement of the crown. Which one of the following options is the main reason for the use of this specific shape of bur when undertaking a crown preparation technique?
   A Can be used interdentally
   B Produces near-parallel preparation
   C Removes caries
   D Removes enamel quickly
   E Unlikely to cause exposure

4. While a permanent crown is being constructed in the laboratory, the dentist will place a temporary crown over the prepared tooth to ensure the patient does not suffer from sensitivity issues in the meantime. Which one of the following options is a material that is not used for temporary crown construction?
   A Aluminium
   B Chromium
   C Plastic
   D Polycarbonate
   E Stainless steel

5. When a tooth is heavily filled or has undergone root canal therapy it is usual to place a crown on it to protect the remaining tooth structure from fracture, thus prolonging the life of the tooth. Various materials are available for crown construction, and that chosen will be guided by aesthetics and function requirements. Which one of the following options is the material that provides a superior 'tooth-like' appearance by mimicking the natural translucency of enamel?
   A All-ceramic
   B Non-precious metal
   C Porcelain bonded
   D Porcelain jacket
   E Yellow gold

6. A bridge is a laboratory-constructed artificial device that is composed of two or more units, one of which is to replace a missing tooth in the dental arch. There are various designs of bridge available to choose from, depending on the individual patient's occlusion and aesthetic requirements. Which one of the following options is a type of bridge that replaces a missing tooth with abutments on just one side of it?
   A Adhesive
   B Fixed-fixed
   C Fixed-moveable
   D Simple cantilever
   E Spring cantilever

7. When a fixed prosthesis is to be cemented into or onto a tooth, the dentist has a wide variety of luting cements to choose from for this purpose. Which one of the following options is an example of a luting cement that holds a prosthesis in place by chemically bonding it to the tooth structure of the abutment tooth?
   A Glass ionomer
   B Light-cure resin
   C Polyester resin
   D Self-cure resin
   E Zinc polycarboxylate

8. Porcelain veneers are fixed prostheses that cover just the labial face of anterior teeth, usually to improve aesthetics. They are cemented in place using special light-cure or dual-cure luting materials, after their fitting surfaces have been air abraded and chemically roughened by the technician to give maximum retention potential. Which one of the following options is the chemical used to roughen the fitting surface of the veneers?
   A Calcium silicate
   B Hydrofluoric acid
   C Hypochlorous acid
   D Phosphoric acid
   E Sodium hypochlorite

9. When patients have several missing teeth they often choose to have a partial denture constructed to replace them to restore their appearance and chewing function. Denture construction involves several stages, the last of which is the fit stage when the completed denture is given to the patient for use. Which one of the following options is an item that may be required for use at the fit appointment?
   A Diamond bur
   B Green stone
   C Rubber cup
   D Stainless steel bur
   E White stone

10. When constructing a set of full dentures for an edentulous patient, the dentist or clinical dental technician must ensure accurate recording of the correct occlusal face height of the patient so that the dentures are comfortable to wear. Which one of the following options is an item that can be used to record the face height of the patient?
   A Bite registration paste
   B Fox plane
   C Le Cron carver
   D Wax rim
   E Willis bite gauge

11. Dentures are removable prostheses, so their retention must be adequate to keep them in position in the mouth during speech and chewing, but weak enough so that the patient can easily remove them for cleaning. Which one of the following options is an aid to functional retention used with partial dentures rather than full dentures?
   A Accurate fit
   B Clasps
   C Natural undercuts
   D Post-dam
   E Suction film

12. When patients have undergone a difficult tooth extraction, they may be left with bony spicules on their ridge that cause discomfort when wearing dentures, as the overlying soft tissues are pressed onto these sharp points when a denture is in place. Which one of the following options is a surgical procedure that can be carried out to remove these sharp bony points?
   A Alveolectomy
   B Alveoplasty
   C Apicectomy
   D Gingivectomy
   E Gingivoplasty

13. Orthodontic appliances are used to align teeth within an arch and align the jaws in relation to each other, so that patients can carry out effective oral hygiene and chew efficiently. Aligning teeth also results in improved aesthetics for the patient and therefore improves their self-esteem in many cases too. Which one of the following options is a type of orthodontic appliance that works by exerting gradual pressure to achieve tooth movement and usually involves several appliances to do so?
   A Aligner
   B Fixed ceramic
   C Fixed metal
   D Functional
   E Removable

14. Orthodontic appliances are used to align teeth within an arch and align the jaws in relation to each other, so that patients can carry out effective oral hygiene and chew efficiently. Aligning teeth also results in improved aesthetics for the patient and therefore improves their self-esteem in many cases too. Which one of the following options is a type of orthodontic appliance that is constructed in a similar way to a partial denture?
   A Aligner
   B Fixed ceramic
   C Fixed metal
   D Removable
   E Retainer

Extended matching questions

For each of the following prosthodontics questions, select the requested number of most appropriate answers from the option list. Each option might be used once, more than once or not at all.

a) Acrylic denture
b) Adhesive bridge
c) Chrome-cobalt denture
d) Conventional bridge
e) Crown former
f) Fixed appliance
g) Implant
h) Obturator
i) Removable appliance
j) Veneer

1. Some patients are unfortunate enough to have congenitally discoloured teeth, due to developmental defects or the action of certain drugs on the enamel as the teeth formed. Several options are available to them for the teeth to be aesthetically improved by the dental team. Which one of the options listed is a device that can be bonded to a discoloured tooth following minimal tooth preparation, to improve its appearance?

2. Missing teeth can be replaced by one of several treatment options available from the dental team. The choice of which is used depends on several factors including patient preference and treatment costs. Which one of the options listed is a tooth replacement option that relies on a titanium prosthesis becoming incorporated into the alveolar bone of the patient, in a process called osseointegration?

3. A patient has attended for advice about replacing her missing upper central incisor teeth, which were extracted several years ago following a car accident. The patient has been wearing an acrylic denture to replace the teeth since then but wishes to discuss alternative options for their replacement with the dentist. Which three of the options listed are the most likely tooth replacements to be discussed with the patient?

Answers

Multiple choice questions

1. *The correct answer is A.* Alginate impressions will shrink if dried, and the resulting casting will be inaccurate. After disinfection they should be wrapped in damp gauze and sealed in an airtight bag for transport to the laboratory, so that the impression remains moist.

2. *The correct answer is B.* Alginate impression material is an irreversible hydrocolloid that is mixed with room temperature water to produce the working mix. The set material is not dimensionally stable and can also tear easily compared to more solid materials. It is therefore not accurate enough to be used for the working models of prosthodontic procedures.

3. *The correct answer is B.* The retention of the crown on the prepared tooth is dependent on the quality of the adhesive used and the near-parallel preparation of the sides of the tooth, giving maximum retention. If the tooth is prepared with the occlusal edge of the sides much narrower than the base, there is minimal mechanical retention and the adhesive alone will have to hold the crown in place. If the occlusal edge of the sides is wider than the base, the crown cannot be seated as undercuts will have been created.

4. *The correct answer is B.* Chromium is a metallic element that is used to construct chrome-cobalt metal dentures. It requires casting at the laboratory and is not a material used in the dental workplace otherwise.

5. *The correct answer is A.* All-ceramic crowns have superior aesthetics to all-metal crowns and to bonded crowns, which have porcelain bonded onto a metallic substructure to appear tooth-like. All-ceramic crowns are also superior to porcelain crowns, as the ceramic zirconia they are made from reflects light better and therefore mimics natural enamel more closely.

6. *The correct answer is D.* This design of bridge removes the likelihood of one of the abutments working loose over time, as tends to happen with fixed-fixed bridges where the abutments are on both sides of the missing tooth. Simple cantilever bridges can be used both anteriorly and posteriorly if sufficient healthy teeth are available as abutments.

7. *The correct answer is D.* The resin used is similar to that of the liquid component of composite restorative materials and the two components chemically set (cure) when mixed together, thus bonding the prosthesis to the tooth. Self-cure resins are usually provided as a double syringe product with a mixing tip that automatically mixes the correct proportions of the two components as they are squeezed out of the syringe.

8. *The correct answer is B.* This is a very strong acid and is usually applied to the fitting surface of the veneer by the technician in the laboratory once it has been formed and before sending the prosthesis to the practice.

9. *The correct answer is D.* The fitting surface of dentures is always checked for any sharp acrylic spicules before they are seated, as they are very uncomfortable for the patient if not removed first. A stainless-steel bur is required to do this. Diamond burs are not used to adjust dentures, stones are used for smoothing and polishing various restoratives and a rubber cup is used during prophylaxis.

10. *The correct answer is E.* The solid top of the measuring gauge is placed under the patient's nose and the moveable bottom under the chin. The moveable piece is then slid up or down into its correct position under the chin, and the measurement between the top and bottom pieces is the face height. This is read off the gauge in mm. When the try-in stage is inserted into the patient's mouth, the face height can be checked with the gauge for the same measurement again.

11. *The correct answer is B.* Metallic clasps can be incorporated into the design of a partial denture when adequate teeth are present in the correct positions and act as 'anchors' for the device. When patients have a full denture, they have no natural teeth remaining so clasps cannot be used to help retain them. All other options can be used to aid retention for both partial and full dentures.

12. *The correct answer is A.* Alveolectomy is a surgical term denoting the surgical removal of all or part of the alveolar bone. Alveoplasty is a surgical term denoting the reshaping of the alveolar bone, usually to improve function such as to create bony undercuts and improve denture retention.

13. *The correct answer is A.* Aligners are produced in sets for the patient to wear in the correct order so that gradual tooth pressure is exerted in a controlled manner until the required tooth movement is achieved. The aligner sets are generated in the laboratory by computer – the pre-treatment study models are scanned in and a 'perfect' end result is created. The computer then designs the set of aligners required to achieve this result, and they are created as three-dimensional print-outs in a plastic material. The correct wearing of the aligner set by the patient is supervised by the dentist.

14. *The correct answer is D.* Removable orthodontic appliances are made of acrylic bases with stainless-steel metal components incorporated for retention (Adam's clasps) and for tooth movements (springs, retractors and so on).

Extended matching questions

1. *The correct answer is j).* Veneers may be constructed in the laboratory from special composite materials or from porcelain or other ceramics and can mask even the darkest discolouration when opaquing materials are used.

2. *The correct answer is g).* The implant is inserted into a precision-drilled hole in the alveolar bone, to the correct size, depth and angulation required. The alveolar bone then gradually grows around the device and into its hollow structure so that it becomes locked into the bone tissue itself by osseointegration.

3. *The correct answers are b), d) and g).* When a patient does not wish to have teeth replaced by a removable option, a denture, then the other options to consider are to place a bridge or one or more implants. Bridges are permanently cemented to one or more suitably prepared, surrounding teeth with the missing teeth incorporated into the design. They can be constructed as adhesive designs with minimal tooth preparation, or as conventional designs with significant tooth preparation. Implants involve no surrounding tooth preparation as they are inserted into the jaw bone in the position of the missing teeth.

11 Extractions and Minor Oral Surgery

Multiple choice questions

1. There are several minor oral surgery procedures that may be carried out in the dental workplace from time to time and for a variety of reasons. Which one of the following options is a procedure that is normally carried out to remove a residual flap of gingiva from the surface of a partially erupted tooth?
   A Alveolectomy
   B Biopsy
   C Flap surgery
   D Gingivectomy
   E Operculectomy

2. Sometimes a patient experiences a complication during or after a minor oral surgery procedure that makes the healing process more prolonged or more complicated. In severe cases that patient may need to undergo further surgery to correct the complication. Which one of the following options is a complication that may occur after a surgical procedure that results in the patient having to reattend that day for an emergency haemostasis procedure requiring sutures?
   A Ankylosis
   B Oroantral fistula
   C Osteitis
   D Reactionary haemorrhage
   E Secondary haemorrhage

3. When a tooth needs to be extracted the dentist may use one or more instruments to carry out the procedure depending on its difficulty. Which one of the following options is an instrument used during the extraction to widen the socket and sever the periodontal ligament attachment?
   A Bayonet forceps
   B Coupland's chisel
   C Cryer's elevator
   D Luxator
   E Warwick James elevator

Questions and Answers for Dental Nurses, Fourth Edition. Carole Hollins.

4. There are various surgical techniques that may be carried out to adjust the shape of the gingivae and aid the patient in maintaining an adequate level of oral hygiene, by allowing more effective removal of plaque. Which one of the following options is a surgical technique performed to reduce the gingival level around a tooth so that more tooth is exposed and available for restoration?
   A Crown lengthening
   B Frenectomy
   C Gingivectomy
   D Gingivoplasty
   E Periodontal flap surgery

5. After patients have undergone an extraction procedure, they should be given written post-operative instructions by the dental team to reduce the risk of any post-operative problems occurring. Which one of the following options is a post-operative instruction that should not be given after an extraction procedure has been carried out?
   A Avoid exercise and alcohol for 24 hours
   B Do not rinse out on day of procedure
   C Do not smoke until sensation has returned
   D Take analgesics if required, except aspirin
   E Use hot saltwater mouthwash after 24 hours

6. Sometimes a tooth cannot be extracted simply but has to be removed by a surgical procedure. Various surgical instruments are available to the dentist to carry out this procedure. Which one of the following options is a surgical instrument used to complete the raising of a mucoperiosteal flap during the surgical extraction of a grossly carious molar tooth?
   A Bone rongeurs
   B Dissecting forceps
   C Kilner retractor
   D Osteotrimmer
   E Periosteal elevator

7. A patient is being assessed for suitability to have several upper right missing teeth replaced by an implant-supported bridge in the area. The teeth have been missing for many years, and radiographs have revealed that alveolar bone resorption in the area has resulted in the maxillary antrum lying close to the bony ridge, making implant placement difficult. Which one of the following options is the term used to describe the particular procedure that may be carried out to correct this problem and allow implants to be placed?
   A Alveolectomy
   B Bone graft
   C Frenectomy
   D Osteotomy
   E Sinus lift

8. Impaction is the term used to describe the situation where a tooth is prevented from fully erupting into the oral cavity by having its path blocked by either bone or another tooth. The tooth remains stuck in its unerupted or partially erupted position within the jaw bone and may cause various problems for the patient in future. Which one of the following options is the term used to describe a tooth that is tilted forwards and become impacted into the tooth next to it?
   A Disto-angular impaction
   B Horizontal impaction
   C Mesio-angular impaction
   D Transverse impaction
   E Vertical impaction

9. The placement of a dental implant is a surgical procedure that involves careful planning and the use of special surgical tools and instruments to create the hole in the alveolar bone for the implant to sit. Which one of the following options is the tool used to create the required depth of hole in the alveolar bone, as predetermined by three-dimensional scans and radiographs?
   A Pilot drill
   B Screw tool
   C Torque ratchet
   D Trephine mill
   E Twist drill

10. There are various surgical techniques that may be carried out to adjust the shape of the gingivae and aid the patient in maintaining an adequate level of oral hygiene, by allowing more effective removal of plaque. Which one of the following options is a surgical technique performed to remove hyperplastic gingivae so that the patient can clean the gingival crevice and interdental areas more thoroughly?
    A Crown lengthening
    B Frenectomy
    C Gingivectomy
    D Gingivoplasty
    E Periodontal flap surgery

11. When a tooth needs to be extracted the dentist may use one or more instruments to carry out the procedure depending on its difficulty. Which one of the following options is an instrument used specifically to extract lower molar teeth, as when used correctly it applies force in the furcation area of the tooth and lifts it out of the socket?
    A Bayonet forceps
    B Coupland's chisel
    C Cowhorn forceps
    D Luxator
    E Winter's elevator

12. Sometimes a patient experiences a complication during or after a minor oral surgery procedure that makes the healing process more prolonged or more complicated. In severe cases that patient may need to undergo further surgery to correct the complication. Which one of the following options is a complication that may occur during a surgical procedure that results in an unnatural connection between the oral cavity and the maxillary sinus?

A Ankylosis
B Oroantral fistula
C Osteitis
D Reactionary haemorrhage
E Secondary haemorrhage

13. When a tooth needs to be extracted the dentist may use one or more instruments to carry out the procedure depending on its difficulty. Which one of the following options is a sharp pointed instrument used during the extraction to engage the side of a curved root and lift it out of the socket in the direction of its curvature, often preventing the need for a full surgical procedure?

A Bayonet forceps
B Coupland's chisel
C Cowhorn forceps
D Cryer's elevator
E Warwick James elevator

Extended matching questions

For each of the following extractions and minor oral surgery questions, select the required number of most appropriate answers from the option list. Each option might be used once, more than once or not at all.

a) Dissecting forceps
b) Handpiece and surgical bur
c) Needle holders
d) Osteotrimmer
e) Periosteal elevator
f) Retractor
g) Scalpel pack
h) Suture pack
i) Suture scissors

1. A patient attended earlier in the day for the extraction of his lower left first molar tooth, which was carried out uneventfully by the dentist. Haemostasis was achieved before the patient was discharged, and full written post-operative instructions were given. Unfortunately, these were ignored and the patient returned to work on a construction site an hour after the extraction. The socket is now bleeding again and the patient is returning to the practice for an emergency appointment. Which three of the options listed are items that are most likely to be required by the dentist to arrest the haemorrhage?

2. A patient is undergoing an alveoplasty procedure to remove the sharp bony edge of her alveolar ridge before having a new denture made, which should then be comfortable to wear. Which one of the options listed is the most likely equipment items to be used to remove the sharp edges of the bone and leave a less jagged ridge?

3. The dentist is carrying out a surgical extraction procedure on an upper molar tooth, and the senior nurse is assisting by providing adequate suction and good patient support by holding the patient's hand, as she is very nervous. You are asked to also assist by holding back the buccal soft tissues to improve access to the surgical field. Which one of the options listed is the most likely item to be used to achieve this?

Answers

Multiple choice questions

1. *The correct answer is E.* The residual flap of gingiva is called the operculum, and the procedure for its complete removal is referred to as an operculectomy. The procedure is often carried out on partially erupted lower third molars, where the operculum is constantly bitten and traumatised by the upper tooth so that the patient has bouts of pericoronitis.
2. *The correct answer is D.* Reactionary haemorrhage occurs within hours of the procedure being carried out and is due to the newly formed blood clot being disturbed or lost from the socket, allowing bleeding to begin again. It usually occurs when the patient has not followed the post-operative instructions correctly, such as by exercising, working, drinking alcohol or washing the mouth out when told not to. It may also occur in patients taking anti-coagulant medications, although this should have been realised and planned for by the dental team before the procedure.
3. *The correct answer is D.* Luxators are hand instruments with a single, sharp, curved blade – either narrow or broad. They are pushed around the top of a root and into the socket, severing the periodontal ligament as they go and widening the socket width so that the tooth or root is effectively pushed up and out of the socket.
4. *The correct answer is A.* This technique is particularly useful in cases where otherwise the height of the tooth available for crown preparation is insufficient for a well-formed and retentive crown to be placed. The amount of gingiva removed cannot exceed that available beyond the junctional attachment, though, as this must be maintained for the health of the periodontium.
5. *The correct answer is C.* Patients should be instructed not to smoke for 24 hours after the procedure, otherwise they risk developing localised osteitis in the bare socket. This is a painful inflammation of the bony walls of the socket that occurs when the blood clot has been disturbed or lost.
6. *The correct answer is E.* The corner of the flap is initially raised using a finer instrument such as the osteotrimmer. Then the periosteal elevator is pushed under the raised corner over the surface of the alveolar bone and towards the root apices, effectively peeling the tissue flap off the bone in the process.
7. *The correct answer is E.* A surgical procedure is carried out to raise the floor of the maxillary antrum (sinus) away from the alveolar ridge so that the depth of bone available for implant placement is increased.
8. *The correct answer is C.* The tooth normally affected is the lower third molar, as they are the last teeth to erupt in the mandible and the space available is limited by the ramus of the mandible. Mesio-angular impactions tend to allow food debris to collect and stagnate distal to the second molar tooth, making both teeth vulnerable to carious attack.

9. *The correct answer is E.* The pilot drill is used to create the guide hole on the alveolar ridge at the exact point where the implant is to be located. This makes a purchase point for the twist drills to engage and gradually create the correct depth of hole for the implant. The depth is checked using a depth gauge that has colour-coded markings that tally with those on the screw tool.

10. *The correct answer is C.* Gingival hyperplasia often occurs in patients prescribed certain medications, especially those to prevent epileptic seizures. The overgrown gingivae makes effective plaque removal very difficult for the patient, and the tissues then become more inflamed still due to the continued presence of the plaque. The tissue is surgically removed using a scalpel or a Blake's gingivectomy knife, with the incision following the contour of the necks of the teeth involved.

11. *The correct answer is C.* Obviously so named because they look like cow's horns, the blades of the forceps are circular with pointed tips that are easily inserted from the buccal and lingual sides of the molar tooth to engage the furcation area. Gentle pressure and squeezing of the forceps' handles together then gradually lifts the tooth out of its socket, often without any additional movements required.

12. *The correct answer is B.* This occurs when upper premolar or molar teeth are being extracted and excessive upwards force on the tooth or root by the dentist causes a perforation of the maxillary sinus. The tooth may still be extracted but leaves a connection between the sinus and the mouth, or in a worst-case scenario the tooth may be pushed into the sinus itself. This then requires hospital intervention to remove the tooth.

13. *The correct answer is D.* These are available as a pair of elevators with the triangular-shaped pointed tip able to engage either the mesial or distal side of a curved root, dependent on whether a left or right tooth is being extracted. They engage even more effectively when a notch is drilled into the root side for a better purchase. Warwick James elevators have rounded tips and are unable to be used in this way.

Extended matching questions

1. *The correct answers are c), h) and i).* The extraction was a simple procedure rather than a surgical one, but the patient has continued to work and caused the wound to begin bleeding again. The dentist will need to place a suture across the socket to apply pressure to the wound edges and stop the bleeding. He will require a suture pack and needle holders to place the suture and suture scissors to trim the ends of the suture material.

2. *The correct answer is b).* The sharp bony edges will be exposed by raising a mucoperiosteal flap off the alveolar ridge, then the sharp edges can be carefully

trimmed with the handpiece and surgical bur and shaped into a more comfortable, rounded ridge before the flap is sutured back into position. Once healing has occurred the new denture can be constructed.

3. *The correct answer is f).* There are various styles of surgical retractor available, and the choice will depend on whether the cheek, the tongue, the lips or a mucoperiosteal flap is to be retracted. During surgical procedures it is very important that adequate retraction is provided by a staff member, especially to avoid injury to the patient.

11a Pain and Anxiety Control

Multiple choice questions

1. Many local anaesthetics are now available for use in dentistry to anaesthetise teeth and their surrounding soft tissues so that treatment can be provided painlessly. They are supplied as glass or plastic cartridges for use in special dental syringes and contain solutions of various components. Which one of the following options is present in the cartridge as a carrying solution for the other constituents and makes up the bulk of the cartridge contents?
   A Anaesthetic
   B Buffering agent
   C Preservative
   D Sterile water
   E Vasoconstrictor

2. When a local anaesthetic is administered before a patient undergoes dental treatment, the injection technique used depends on the anatomical location of the sensory nerves supplying the area and the tooth to be treated. Which one of the following options is the injection technique that involves depositing the local anaesthetic solution into the spongy bone of the jaw via a small hole drilled through the cortical plate of the alveolar bone?
   A Infiltration injection
   B Intraligamentary injection
   C Intraosseous injection
   D Nerve block
   E Topical

3. Some patients experience high levels of anxiety when having to undergo dental treatment and require some form of anxiety control technique to enable them to do so. Younger patients may also require anxiety control when undergoing unpleasant dental procedures, such as extractions. Which one of the following options is an anxiety control technique that uses a mixture of gases breathed in through the nose to provide conscious sedation?

Questions and Answers for Dental Nurses, Fourth Edition. Carole Hollins.

A Inhalation sedation
B Intranasal sedation
C Multi-drug intravenous sedation
D Oral sedation
E Single-drug intravenous sedation

4. When administering a local anaesthetic to a patient the dental team must ensure that they avoid an inoculation injury, where someone other than the patient is pierced by the used local anaesthetic needle. Which one of the following options is an action that will not prevent a staff member from suffering an inoculation injury?
A Only clinician handles equipment
B Use 'safety' syringe with slide cover
C Use needle guard device
D Use re-sheathing device
E Wear appropriate PPE

5. During an intravenous sedation procedure, the suitably trained dental nurse assists the dentist by regularly monitoring the patient both manually and with the use of a pulse oximeter machine. Which one of the following options is a monitored vital sign that may alter if the patient is given an overdose of the sedation drug midazolam?
A Blood pressure
B Breathing rate
C Oxygen saturation
D Pulse quality
E Pulse rate

6. When a local anaesthetic is administered before a patient undergoes dental treatment, the injection technique used depends on the anatomical location of the sensory nerves supplying the area and the tooth to be treated. Which one of the following options is the injection technique that involves depositing the local anaesthetic solution under the surface of the oral soft tissues and against a nerve trunk as it enters or emerges from the alveolar bone of the jaws?
A Infiltration injection
B Intraligamentary injection
C Intraosseous injection
D Nerve block
E Topical

7. The dental team has access to several different types of local anaesthetic solutions for use when carrying out dental treatment, each with various constituents making up the solution itself. Which one of the following options is the constituent that is present in some types of local anaesthetic to prolong the length of time that the clinician may provide treatment painlessly?

A Anaesthetic
B Buffering agent
C Preservative
D Sterile water
E Vasoconstrictor

8. Some patients experience high levels of anxiety when having to undergo dental treatment and require some form of anxiety control technique to enable them to do so. Younger patients may also require anxiety control when undergoing unpleasant dental procedures, such as extractions. Which one of the following options is an anxiety control technique that is usually only used when other techniques cannot be, as the depth of sedation produced is unpredictable and cannot be controlled by the sedationist?
   A Inhalation sedation
   B Intranasal sedation
   C Multi-drug intravenous sedation
   D Oral sedation
   E Single-drug intravenous sedation

9. The dental team have access to several different types of local anaesthetic preparations, and although their use is often based on personal preference by the clinician, some have various constituents that make them unsafe for use in certain categories of patients. Which one of the following options is a type of local anaesthetic that is not recommended for use in pregnant women due to its Octapressin content?
   A Articaine
   B Lignocaine 2%
   C Mepivacaine 3%
   D Prilocaine 3%
   E Prilocaine 4%

10. One of the conscious sedation techniques available for use by the dental team is that of inhalation sedation, where the patient is sedated using a controlled mixture of oxygen and nitrous oxide through a nasal hood. Which one of the following options is the colour of a nitrous oxide gas cylinder?
    A Black
    B Black with white shoulder
    C Blue
    D Blue with white shoulder
    E White

11. When a local anaesthetic is administered before a patient undergoes dental treatment, the injection technique used depends on the anatomical location of the sensory nerves supplying the area and the tooth to be treated. Which one of the following options is the injection technique that involves depositing the

local anaesthetic solution under the surface of the oral soft tissues and outside the alveolar bone of the jaws?

A Infiltration injection
B Intraligamentary injection
C Intraosseous injection
D Nerve block
E Topical

Extended matching questions

For each of the following pain and anxiety control questions, select the single most appropriate answer from the option list. Each option might be used once, more than once or not at all.

a) Acupuncture
b) Aspirating technique
c) Hypnosis
d) Infiltration technique
e) Inhalation sedation
f) Intraligamentary technique
g) Intraosseous technique
h) Intravenous sedation
i) Nerve block technique

1. A patient is to undergo a crown preparation on her lower right first molar tooth, and the dentist is about to administer a local anaesthetic to ensure the procedure is painless. Which one of the options listed is the technique the dentist will use to ensure that the local anaesthetic solution is deposited correctly around the nerve, rather than injected into a blood vessel by mistake?

2. A patient is undergoing a surgical extraction of a lower second molar tooth that is grossly carious. Unfortunately, the procedure is proving very painful as the tooth appears not to be sufficiently anaesthetised, and the dentist suspects there may be an abscess present. Which one of the options listed is an additional technique the dentist can use to administer local anaesthetic directly into the periodontium of the tooth and provide sufficient anaesthesia for the procedure to be completed?

3. A healthy young adult patient has decided to proceed with an implant procedure to replace his upper central incisor teeth, which were extracted following an injury while playing rugby. The teeth were extracted while he was a teenager and unfortunately it was a painful experience and the patient is now anxious about further surgery. Which one of the options listed is the most likely technique to be recommended by the dentist to ensure the patient is sufficiently relaxed, calm and unaware of proceedings during and after the procedure to place the implants?

Answers

Multiple choice questions

1. *The correct answer is D.* The water is sterile so that it does not react with any of the other constituents and also prevents contamination of the cartridge contents by any water-borne micro-organisms.
2. *The correct answer is C.* This technique is useful when anaesthetising lower molar teeth and inferior dental nerve blocks have failed previously, often due to the nerve lying in an unusual position. The kit contains the bore drills for penetrating the cortical plate, which can be used with a conventional slow-speed handpiece. The needles provided are exactly the same size as the drills and are used with a conventional local anaesthetic syringe to deposit the solution.
3. *The correct answer is A.* A controlled mixture of oxygen and nitrous oxide gases is inhaled through a nasal hood by the patient to provide an adequate level of conscious sedation for dental treatment to be carried out by the clinician. The technique is particularly useful for younger patients and those with certain medical conditions that make intravenous sedation riskier for them.
4. *The correct answer is E.* Local anaesthetic needles are very sharp and will pierce through any style of gloves used in the dental workplace, even household gloves worn during decontamination procedures. PPE provides no protection against inoculation injuries; instead they should be prevented by the use of one of the safety devices listed and by the equipment being handled by the clinician only and not passed from nurse to clinician and back again after use.
5. *The correct answer is B.* Midazolam causes a reduction in the rate and depth of respiration in many patients, but an overdose of the drug can result in severe respiratory depression. In these situations, the patient's airway must be supported by the dental team using an airway device until breathing returns to normal, otherwise the patient may go into respiratory arrest.
6. *The correct answer is D.* In particular, the inferior dental nerve is anaesthetised with this technique, either completely by the administration of a nerve block as the nerve trunk is about to enter the mandible through the mandibular foramen, or just the terminal section of the nerve as it emerges from the mandible through the mental foramen.
7. *The correct answer is E.* Vasoconstrictors are drugs that act to close, or constrict, blood vessels so that the blood supply to the area is reduced. This slows down the rate at which the local anaesthetic is removed from the area and taken to the liver to be detoxified, thereby prolonging the length of time that the area is numb. This allows the clinician more time to provide dental treatment and is especially useful for long procedures such as endodontics, prosthodontic preparations and surgical procedures.

8. *The correct answer is D.* With this technique the patient is given a relatively large oral dose of a sedative drug, usually midazolam, while at the dental workplace and by the dentist. The patient is required to take the drug on the premises so that the response and level of sedation can be witnessed and monitored by the staff. Various factors affect the depth of sedation achieved, including the speed with which the drug is absorbed from the stomach and the amount of body fat the patient has.

9. *The correct answer is D.* Octapressin is a drug used in childbirth that stimulates the muscles of the womb to contract. Although it is present in small amounts in certain local anaesthetics and acts as a vasoconstrictor, there is a potential for the drug to act on a pregnant patient's womb and cause her to go into premature labour.

10. *The correct answer is C.* Both the cylinder and all of the pipework carrying nitrous oxide to the inhalation machine are coloured blue to ensure it is not mistaken for the oxygen supply. Oxygen cylinders are coloured black with a white shoulder and the pipework is white.

11. *The correct answer is A.* An infiltration technique is used to anaesthetise sensory nerves that lie superficial to the alveolar bones of the jaws and can be used to anaesthetise all of the upper teeth and surrounding soft tissues and the lower incisor teeth and surrounding soft tissues.

Extended matching questions

1. *The correct answer is b).* A nerve block technique will be used to deliver the local anaesthetic but, once the needle has been positioned and before injecting, the dentist will draw back on the syringe handle to see if any blood is drawn into the cartridge. If any appears it indicates that a blood vessel has been pierced, so the needle needs to be repositioned before injecting. This is called the aspirating technique.

2. *The correct answer is f).* A ligmaject syringe is used to deliver one or more additional cartridges directly into the periodontal ligament space and provide a greater depth of anaesthesia to the tooth. A normal local anaesthetic cartridge and short needle are sufficient but the special 'gun-type' device must be used, as it has a protective sheath around the cartridge to protect the patient if it cracks. Considerable pressure is usually required to deposit the anaesthetic solution into the ligament.

3. *The correct answer is h).* One of the benefits of providing dental treatment under intravenous sedation is that the drug usually used, midazolam, causes amnesia so no matter how difficult the treatment proves to be, the patient will never remember any of the proceedings. This is extremely useful in encouraging irregular attenders to become regular patients, as they know if treatment is required they will not recall anything. Also, by attending regularly the dental team can prevent problems arising initially or intervene at an early stage to minimise the level of treatment required.

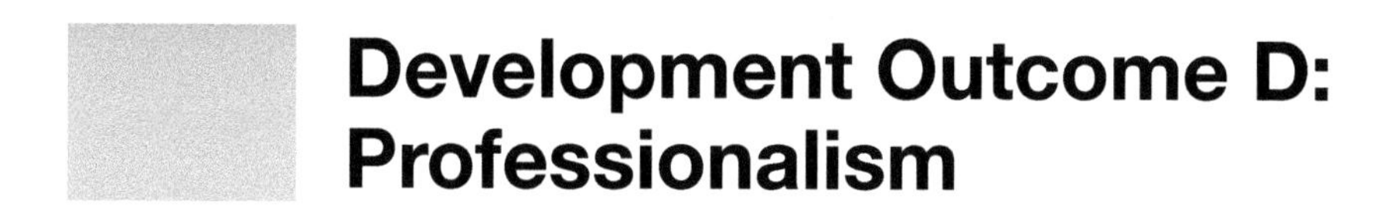

Development Outcome D: Professionalism

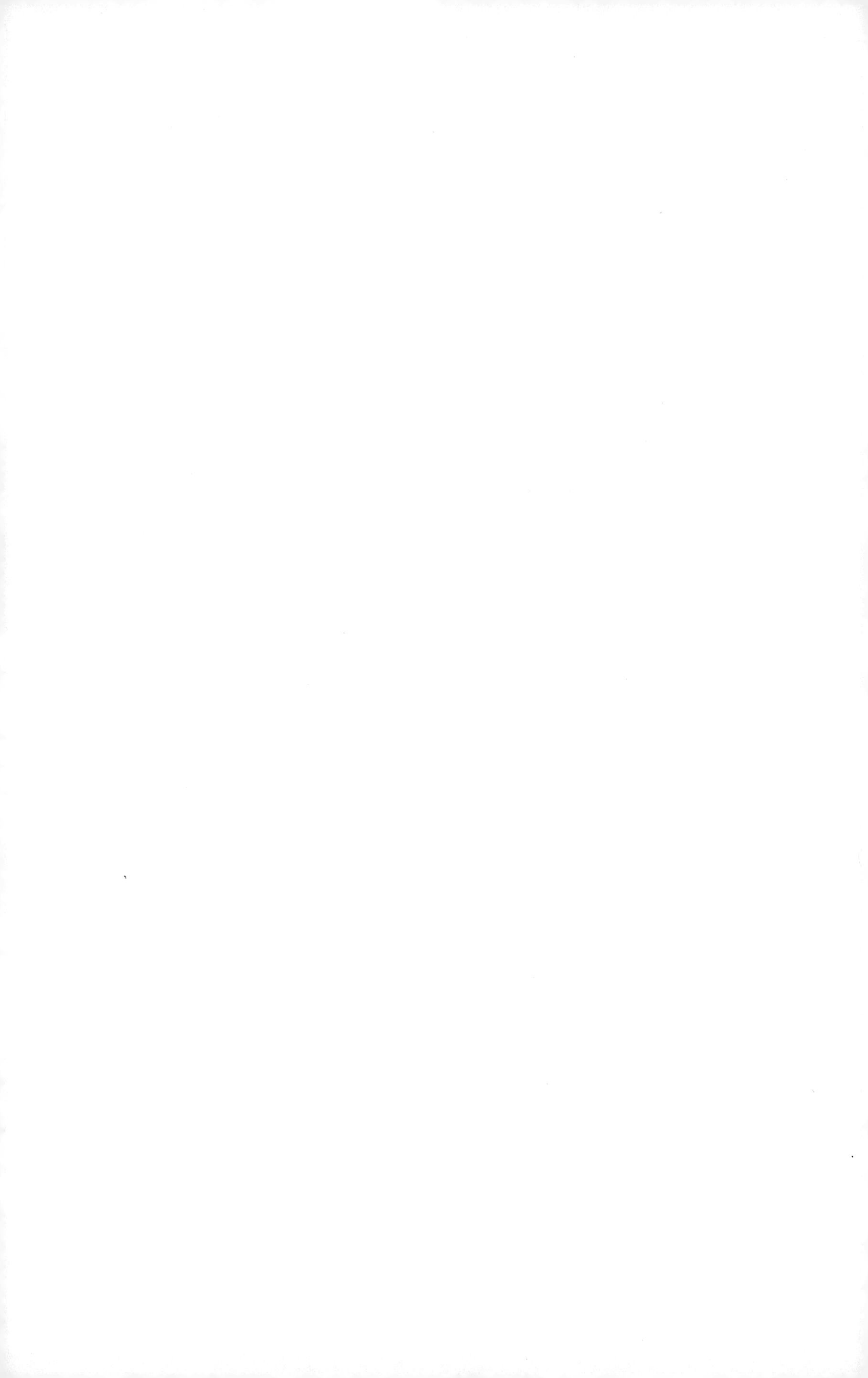

12 GDC Standards and Equality and Diversity

Multiple choice questions

1. All General Dental Council (GDC) registrants are expected to abide by various professional obligations during their working career, one of which is always to ensure their professional activities follow the guidance within the GDC publication *Scope of Practice*. Which one of the following options enshrines this obligation?
   A Be able to demonstrate their fitness to practise
   B Ensure that all patients have equal rights
   C Maintain their professional registration
   D Undertake lifelong learning in their areas of competence
   E Work within their professional level of competence

2. The General Dental Council publication *Standards for the Dental Team* sets out the nine ethical principles to be followed by all team members in relation to professionalism and practice. Which one of the following options is the numbered principle that gives information about the standards of behaviour expected in relation to data security?
   A Communicate effectively with patients (2)
   B Have a clear and effective complaints procedure (5)
   C Maintain and protect patients' information (4)
   D Obtain valid consent (3)
   E Raise concerns if patients are at risk (8)

3. The requirement for the dental team to be appropriately trained and qualified is enshrined in the General Dental Council (GDC) Standards document. Which one of the following options is the specific core ethical principle of professionalism in this document that deals with the issue of maintaining and updating skills and knowledge?
   A Principle 1
   B Principle 3
   C Principle 5

Questions and Answers for Dental Nurses, Fourth Edition. Carole Hollins.

D Principle 7
E Principle 9

4. Completion of continuing professional development activities is a requirement by the General Dental Council (GDC) for all registrants. The previous 'core topics' are now referred to as 'highly recommended topics' and have been identified by the GDC as relevant to almost all registrant groups. Which one of the following options is the 'highly recommended topic' that must be completed on an annual basis by all registrants?
   A Complaints handling
   B Medical emergencies
   C Oral cancer and early detection
   D Radiography and radiation protection
   E Safeguarding children and young adults

5. Annual reviews in the form of staff appraisals provide evidence of good practice in the workplace by the employer and should be carried out in all dental workplaces. Usually, they cover several areas of appraisal in one session unless an issue has been highlighted that requires specific review and discussion. Which one of the following options is an area of appraisal that should review a staff member's patient management skills?
   A Administration
   B Clinical
   C Communication
   D Development
   E Teamwork

6. Annual reviews in the form of staff appraisals provide evidence of good practice in the workplace by the employer and should be carried out in all dental workplaces. Usually, they cover several areas of appraisal in one session unless an issue has been highlighted that requires specific review and discussion. Which one of the following options is an area of appraisal that should demonstrate a staff member's acceptance of authority within the workplace?
   A Administration
   B Clinical
   C Communication
   D Development
   E Teamwork

7. In 2018 the General Dental Council introduced the enhanced continuing professional development scheme (eCPD) for all registrants, to assist them in maintaining and updating their skills, knowledge and competencies in a more effective manner than the old-style CPD scheme. Which one of the following

options is a requirement of eCPD that allows the registrant to self-evaluate and reflect on training needs throughout the 5-year CPD cycle?

A Activity log
B Lifelong learning
C Personal development plan
D Quality assurance
E SWOT analysis

8. In 2018 the General Dental Council (GDC) introduced the enhanced continuing professional development scheme (eCPD) for all registrants, to assist them in maintaining and updating their skills, knowledge and competencies in a more effective manner than the old-style CPD scheme. Which one of the following options is a requirement of eCPD that enables registrants to provide evidence of their completed CPD activities in relation to the GDC's development outcomes?

A Activity log
B Lifelong learning
C Personal development plan
D Quality assurance
E SWOT analysis

9. A personal development plan (PDP) should be used by registrants to identify their own continuing professional development needs in relation to the General Dental Council's development outcomes. Which one of the following options is a tool that can be used when developing the PDP to determine any factors that may be preventing registrants from achieving their goals?

A Activity log
B Field of practice
C Lifelong learning
D Quality assurance
E SWOT analysis

10. SMART (as in SMART objectives) is an acronym used in education that helps users to focus their efforts when considering their career development pathway and how to achieve their desired or required goals. In this context it makes the registrant's personal development plan achievable. Which one of the following options is the term from the acronym that implies the end goal must be within the reach of that particular registrant?

A Attainable
B Measurable
C Realistic
D Specific
E Time-based

11. Within the dental workplace, various compliance and good governance requirements should be in place that enable the team to assess the quality and effectiveness of certain areas of the service they deliver to their patients. Which one of the following options is the term used for an individual governance procedure that aims to examine a service area to verify whether set standards are being achieved or not?
    - A Appraisal
    - B Audit
    - C Inspection
    - D Lifelong learning
    - E Peer review

12. To discriminate against someone is to be prejudiced and treat them differently and unfavourably from others on the grounds of their personal traits, beliefs or abilities. Which one of the following options is the type of discrimination shown when a patient is not offered a certain type of dental treatment because it is believed they cannot afford to pay for it?
    - A Age discrimination
    - B Disability discrimination
    - C Racial/ethnic discrimination
    - D Religious discrimination
    - E Socioeconomic discrimination

13. To discriminate against someone is to be prejudiced and treat them differently and unfavourably from others on the grounds of their personal traits, beliefs or abilities. Which one of the following options is the type of discrimination shown when an employer advertises a new position for a dental hygienist at the workplace and sets a preferred age range for all applicants?
    - A Age discrimination
    - B Disability discrimination
    - C Racial/ethnic discrimination
    - D Religious discrimination
    - E Socioeconomic discrimination

14. To discriminate against someone is to be prejudiced and treat them differently and unfavourably from others on the grounds of their personal traits, beliefs or abilities. Which one of the following options is the type of discrimination shown when a deaf patient is unable to receive dental treatment because staff refuse to lower their face masks to allow him to lip read?
    - A Age discrimination
    - B Disability discrimination
    - C Racial/ethnic discrimination
    - D Religious discrimination
    - E Socioeconomic discrimination

Extended matching questions

For each of the following GDC standards and equality and diversity questions, select the single most appropriate answer from the option list. Each option might be used once, more than once or not at all.

a) Dignity and respect
b) Direct age discrimination
c) Disability discrimination
d) Equal opportunities
e) Equality and diversity
f) Harassment
g) Honesty and integrity
h) Indirect sex discrimination
i) Victimisation

1. An elderly patient has attended for treatment to provide a new set of full dentures but is struggling to understand the dental nurse's instructions to remove his old dentures because he is hard of hearing. The dental staff are all wearing masks so the patient is unable to lip read, as he usually does. After several minutes the dentist leaves the surgery and refuses to treat the patient as she believes he is 'a time waster'. Which one of the options listed is the type of discrimination shown by the dentist towards the patient in this scenario?

2. Principle 1 of the GDC Standards document states that all registrants should 'put patients' interests first' and that they therefore have a duty of care towards their patients to always act in their best interests. This includes taking a patient's preferences into account and being sensitive to their individual needs and values, even if they differ from those of the registrant. Which one of the options listed is the phrase used to describe the values the GDC expect a registrant to show towards patients in this respect?

3. A well-led dental workplace should ensure that all its staff and patients are treated in the same way and as individuals, regardless of ethnicity, nationality, gender, age, disability or socioeconomic class. Which one of the options listed is the term used to describe this principle?

4. A young dentist who joined the practice 6 months ago has approached the business owner to complain about the behaviour of the practice manager towards him. The dentist says she often tells jokes during the lunch hour which he finds upsetting and offensive as they are usually defamatory towards Asians. He also says the manager is often unhelpful towards him and refused to show him how to use the computer software when he first arrived. Which one of the options listed is the term used to describe the behaviour of the practice manager towards the dentist?

5. The dental workplace has a vacancy for a new dental nurse and has placed an advert in the local newspaper for applicants to contact the practice to arrange interviews. The employer oversees the application process and disregards two candidates because they are both in their 40s, and he believes they will not have long-term plans to stay in the profession. Which one of the options listed is the equality issue that has been raised by the employer?

6. Principle 1 of the GDC Standards document states the overarching principle of putting patients' interests first at all times, so that the dental team always put the best interests of the patient before those of financial gain and business need. Which one of the options listed is the phrase used to describe the values the GDC expect registrants to adhere to, to achieve this?

Answers

Multiple choice questions

1. *The correct answer is E.* This publication gives information about the additional skills that each registrant group may achieve, after qualification, following a period of suitable training. It is particularly informative for those dental nurses wishing to broaden their career by undertaking extended duties or post-registration qualifications.

2. *The correct answer is C.* Patients have a right to expect that their personal and clinical information held by the dental workplace will be kept secure at all times and will only be divulged to third parties in line with current data security legislation.

3. *The correct answer is D.* The GDC expect all members of the dental team to ensure that their knowledge and skills are kept up to date at all times – this is the core principle of continuing professional development and enshrines the idea of lifelong learning.

4. *The correct answer is B.* Any member of the dental team may be present at the time of a medical emergency, whether in the workplace or not. They may be the only person present and must be able to provide effective basic life support alone until others arrive. The medical emergency may even involve a senior colleague – the person who all assumed would take control and lead the team if ever there was an emergency, and who now needs someone else to take charge and maintain their life. It is imperative that every team member has annual refresher training and hands-on practice at basic life support.

5. *The correct answer is C.* Good communication skills are essential when dealing with patients. Without them, patients cannot understand what advice is being given, what treatment is being proposed, what that treatment involves, what the risks and benefits and alternatives are and so on. Also, the manner of communication used is most important – patients do not respond well to inarticulate, dismissive or rude staff, and poor communication skills form the basis of many, many complaints against members of the dental team.

6. *The correct answer is E.* Effective teamwork involves several people working together safely and in harmony to provide an efficient service for their patients. This includes the acceptance of the hierarchy within the workplace and the authority of the senior person with overall responsibility for the team and their actions.

7. *The correct answer is C.* The personal development plan should be developed by team members to determine if they have gaps in their knowledge or skills or require updates in any of their competencies. It should be used as a living document that is continually added to throughout the cycle and then rolled over into the next CPD cycle as necessary.

8. *The correct answer is A.* The activity log is effectively a register of all of the enhanced CPD activities and events that the registrant has undertaken and completed throughout the cycle. It should contain the title and description of the activity, the date undertaken, number of hours of CPD claimed and the GDC development outcomes that each activity relates to. There must also be corresponding evidence available for each activity to prove that it meets the criteria for being verifiable (such as a certificate of participation).

9. *The correct answer is E.* A SWOT analysis identifies any personal issues that may be helping (Strengths) or hindering (Weaknesses) the registrant, and also any external factors that may be of use (Opportunities) or not (Threats) when considering how to achieve goals.

10. *The correct answer is A.* There must be a realistic pathway open to registrants to enable them to achieve their objectives. For example, if the registrant is a dental nurse and wishes to train to become a dental therapist, they must meet the University entrance requirements and receive the offer of a place there, they must have sufficient funds to complete the course as it involves full-time training and there must be a realistic prospect of securing a job once qualified.

11. *The correct answer is B.* Audits are carried out by an individual looking at a specific topic of the service provided to patients. They can be clinical or non-clinical; either way the aim is to determine whether the techniques used under examination are effective or not. If not, then improvements can be made and the topic re-examined at a later date to ensure the quality is being maintained or improved further.

12. *The correct answer is E.* A patient from a low socioeconomic background may be assumed to be unable to afford molar endodontic treatment, for example, so the option is not offered when being discussed with the dental team and the tooth is extracted instead. This is completely discriminatory and would form the basis of a litigation complaint against the team member, as informed consent had not been given by the patient for the extraction.

13. *The correct answer is A.* A younger team member may be desirable for the employer and their wishes for longevity of service and the achievement of a having a young team, but older applicants outside the preferred age range cannot be refused for employment consideration simply because of their age. Apart from being discriminatory, they may be more experienced and better qualified than younger applicants anyway.

14. *The correct answer is B.* Even during the coronavirus pandemic of 2020–2021 when the wearing of masks everywhere became mandatory for all, dental teams found ways of overcoming this issue and providing suitable care as required. Visors were worn without masks while socially distancing and discussing treatment with deaf patients so they could lip read. Fit-tested hood devices were also available with full facial exposure so that deaf patients

could receive dental treatment safely. Before the coronavirus pandemic there was no excuse for not lowering a mask to communicate effectively with deaf patients and those who were hard of hearing.

Extended matching questions

1. *The correct answer is c).* The patient is being treated less favourably because of his partial deafness, and the staff have failed to recognise the problem. Simply lowering their masks while still social distancing would have allowed the patient to understand what he was being asked to do. The dental team also exhibited poor communication skills in this scenario.
2. *The correct answer is a).* Standard 1.2 states that registrants should 'treat every patient with dignity and respect at all times'. Differences in opinion about religion, political beliefs and so on should not change the way a patient is dealt with or treated by a registrant. Nervous and anxious patients, older patients who take more time to move around the premises and so on all must be shown dignity and respect for their individual circumstances by the registrant.
3. *The correct answer is d).* No-one should be treated differently, especially less favourably, because of a difference from others for any of these reasons. To do so is to discriminate against them.
4. *The correct answer is f).* Harassment is a type of discrimination where a person is picked on and made to feel uncomfortable by others because of their sex, race, age, disability or religion. It may involve action, behaviour, comments or physical contact that is found objectionable, offensive or intimidating by the recipient. The recipient may feel humiliated, threatened or patronised by the actions or behaviour of the perpetrator.
5. *The correct answer is b).* The two candidates have been discriminated against because of their age. Direct age discrimination is to treat someone less favourably on the grounds of their age – in this scenario the employer assumes the older candidates will not remain in the job role as long as a younger candidate may.
6. *The correct answer is g).* Standard 1.3 states that registrants should 'be honest and act with integrity'. They should not overstate their professional skills by advertising themselves as 'specialists' so that patients are misled, or bring the profession into disrepute. The trust that patients and colleagues have for a registrant must be justified at all times, and this is achieved by always acting honestly and adhering to a high moral code.

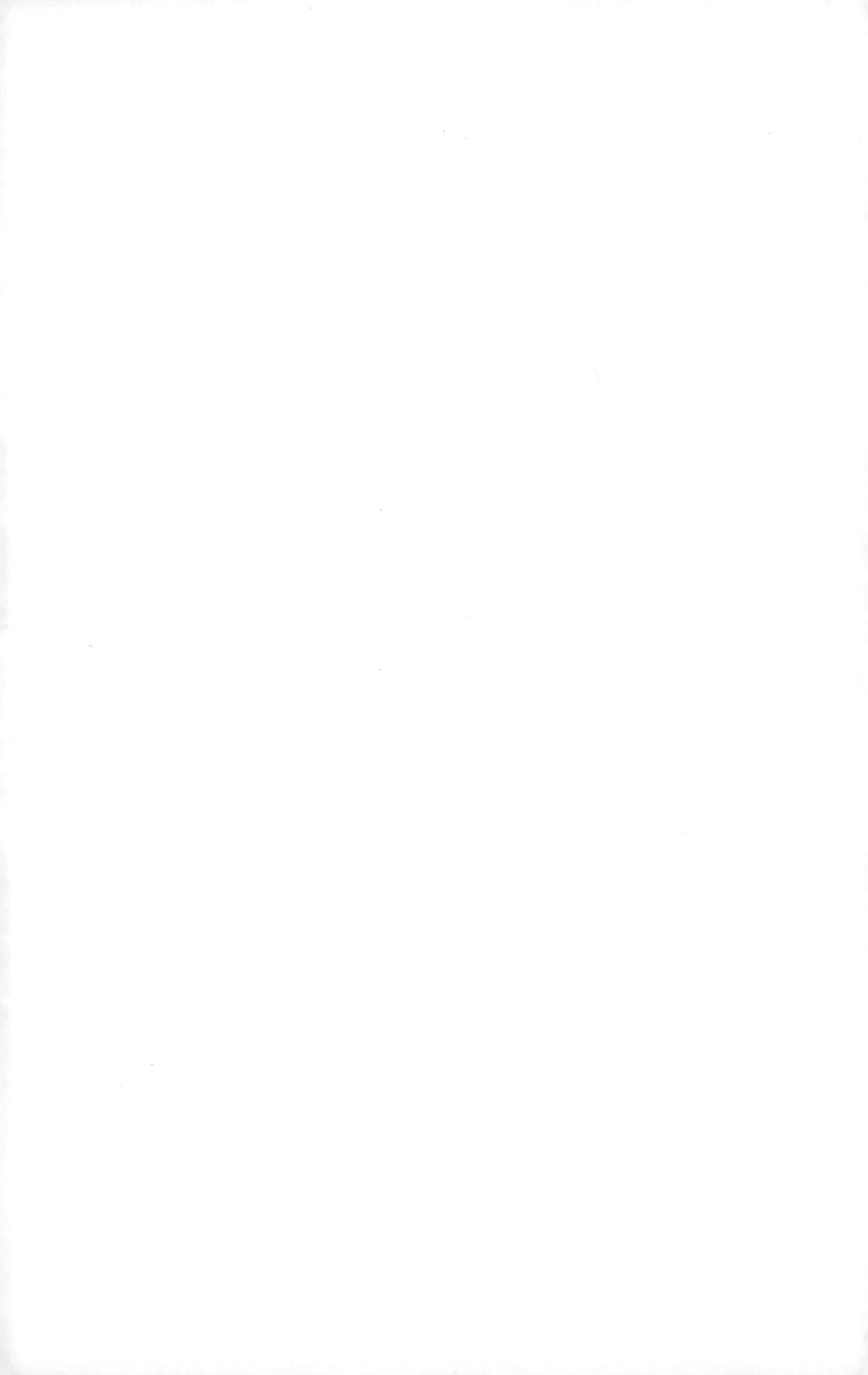

13 Legal and Ethical Issues

Multiple choice questions

1. Dental workplaces have the potential to be dangerous places for both staff and patients if the regulations and legislation governing their safe operation are ignored or flouted. It is important that all staff are familiar with the health and safety aspects of their workplace and their own duties and that they receive regular updates and training as necessary. Which one of the following options is the guidance available for staff to follow in relation to the safe use and decontamination of DUWLs in the workplace?
   A HTM 01-05
   B HTM 03-01
   C HTM 04-01
   D HTM 07-01
   E RIDDOR

2. All workplaces are legally required to be compliant with Health and Safety at Work legislation. Health and safety issues in the dental workplace cover an array of other regulations and codes of conduct that must be adhered to under the Health and Safety Act. Which one of the following options is a set of regulations ensuring that workers are aware of the types of personal protective equipment that should be available for their use while in the workplace?
   A Hazardous Waste Regulations 2005
   B Ionising Radiation (Medical Exposures) Regulations 2017
   C Ionising Radiation Regulations 2017
   D Personal Protective Equipment at Work Regulations 1992
   E Water Supply (Water Fittings) Regulations 1999

3. The GDC publishes various documents and guidance notes that provide invaluable information to all members of the dental team about their professional duties and the standards expected of them by both the regulator and the public. Which one of the following publications gives information about the nine

Questions and Answers for Dental Nurses, Fourth Edition. Carole Hollins.

ethical principles of practice to which all students and registrants are expected to adhere?

A *Preparing for Practice*
B *Scope of Practice*
C *Standards for the Dental Team*
D *Student Professionalism and Fitness to Practice*
E *The First Five Years*

4. The vast majority of dental workplaces use ionising radiation techniques to aid diagnosis and treatment of their patients. The workplaces must all abide by the necessary legislation involved and each appoint a person to ensure that all staff members comply with the policies and protocols in place for patient and staff safety. Which one of the following options is the title of this appointed person?

A Clinical lead
B Legal person
C Medical physics expert
D Radiation protection advisor
E Radiation protection supervisor

5. The General Dental Council learning outcomes have been developed so that a student who achieves them will be able to practise safely, effectively and professionally as a registrant. Which one of the following options is the term used to describe the underpinning, theoretical information that a student must gain to show understanding of a particular subject?

A Attitudes
B Behaviours
C Competence
D Knowledge
E Skills

6. All registered members of the dental team are governed by various Acts and Orders of Parliament, many of which are in place to keep their patients and the public safe. Which one of the following options is the legislation that requires all team members to have security in place against harm, loss or liability while working as a General Dental Council registrant?

A Dentists' Act 1984 (Amendment Order 2005)
B Health and Safety at Work Act 1974
C Health and Social Care Act 2008
D Health Care and Associated Professions (Indemnity Arrangements) Order 2014
E Management of Health and Safety at Work Regulations 1999

7. All registered members of the dental team are governed by various Acts and Orders of Parliament, many of which are in place to keep their patients and the public safe. Which one of the following options is the legislation that legally enables a person to call themselves a dental nurse, once they have achieved a suitable qualification and become registered with the General Dental Council?

A Dentists' Act 1984 (Amendment Order 2005)
B Health and Safety at Work Act 1974
C Health and Social Care Act 2008
D Health Care and Associated Professions (Indemnity Arrangements) Order 2014
E Management of Health and Safety at Work Regulations 1999

8. The General Dental Council stipulate that a dental professional's duty of care is to always put the patient's interests first and act to protect them. This applies to both students and registrants, and once qualified all members of the dental team are expected to uphold their professional obligations. Which one of the following options is the requirement to always strive to update and improve their level of knowledge in their chosen field?
A Demonstrate fitness to practise
B Maintain professional registration
C Show equality, respect diversity
D Undertake lifelong learning
E Work within scope of practice

9. All workplaces are legally required to be compliant with Health and Safety at Work legislation. Health and safety issues in the dental workplace cover an array of other regulations and codes of conduct that must be adhered to under the Health and Safety Act. Which one of the following options is a set of regulations ensuring that workers are not adversely affected by using computers for long periods while at work?
A COSHH
B Health and Safety (Display Screen Equipment) Regulations 1992
C Health and Safety (First Aid) Regulations 1981
D Pressure Systems Safety Regulations 2000
E RIDDOR

10. Full compliance with health and safety legislation in the dental workplace involves following a large range of regulations, orders and health technical memorandums. Which one of the options listed is the set of regulations to be followed in the event of an outbreak of Legionella on the premises?
A COSHH 2002
B Health and Safety (First Aid) Regulations 1981
C Personal Protective Equipment at Work Regulations 1992
D RIDDOR 2013
E Water Supply (Water Fittings) Regulations 1999

11. Dental workplaces have the potential to be dangerous places for both staff and patients if the regulations and legislation governing their safe operation are ignored or flouted. It is important that all staff are familiar with the health and safety aspects of their workplace and their own duties and that they receive regular updates and training as necessary. Which one of the following options is the guidance available for staff to follow in relation to infection prevention and control in the workplace?

A HTM 01-05
B HTM 03-01
C HTM 04-01
D HTM 07-01
E RIDDOR

12. Dental workplaces have the potential to be dangerous places for both staff and patients if the regulations and legislation governing their safe operation are ignored or flouted. It is important that all staff are familiar with the health and safety aspects of their workplace and their own duties and that they receive regular updates and training as necessary. Which one of the following options is the guidance available for staff to follow in relation to the correct segregation and disposal of hazardous waste from the workplace?
    A HTM 01-05
    B HTM 03-01
    C HTM 04-01
    D HTM 07-01
    E RIDDOR

13. Dental workplaces have the potential to be dangerous places for both staff and patients if the regulations and legislation governing their safe operation are ignored or flouted. It is important that all staff are familiar with the health and safety aspects of their workplace and their own duties and that they receive regular updates and training as necessary. Which one of the following options is the guidance available for staff to follow in relation to the explosion of an autoclave in the dental workplace?
    A HTM 01-05
    B HTM 03-01
    C HTM 04-01
    D HTM 07-01
    E RIDDOR

Extended matching questions

For each of the following legal and ethical questions, select the required number of most appropriate answers from the option list. Each option might be used once, more than once or not at all.

a) COSHH
b) HTM 01-05
c) HTM 04-01
d) HTM 07-01
e) IR(ME)R17

f) IRR17
g) *Preparing for Practice*
h) RIDDOR
i) *Scope of Practice*
j) *Standards for the Dental Team*

1. A new associate dentist has joined the practice and is keen to begin offering Botox treatments to his patients, as an additional source of revenue for the workplace. The treatment has never been carried out on the premises before, and the business owner is unsure whether additional hazardous waste receptacles are required or if the used syringes can be disposed of in the yellow sharps bin. Which one of the options listed is the document that will provide information about the issue?

2. A busy dental workplace has four dental surgeries operating 5 days a week, each with its own intra-oral X-ray machine installed for use. The surgeries are of different sizes and layouts, so the required details of the 2 metre safety zone vary in each. Which one of the options listed is the set of regulations concerned with the drawing up of a contingency plan for each of the surgeries, in the event of a malfunction of the X-ray machine within it?

3. A member of staff who normally carries out all of the infection control and prevention duties at the workplace is on holiday, and one of her colleagues has been asked to carry out the foil ablation test on the ultrasonic bath. Which one of the options listed is a document that should provide the colleague with the information required to carry out the test correctly?

4. Following a successful interview for the position of practice manager at a newly opened dental practice, a senior dental nurse is concerned that her new work contract contains a 'gagging clause' that would restrict her ability to raise a concern if she felt the need to do so in the future. Which one of the options listed is a document that the nurse should consult to gain further information about the issue?

5. During a restorative procedure to place a composite filling in a tooth, the dentist accidentally spills a drop of acid etchant onto the patient's lower lip. The area is under local anaesthetic so the patient is unaware, but her lip is marked despite the etchant being wiped off with a tissue. Which one of the options listed is a document folder that should detail the first aid actions that can be taken by the dental team to reduce the severity of any injury?

6. A new member of staff has been asked to carry out the monthly temperature checks on the water outlets in the dental workplace and record the findings,

using the appropriate documentation, in the 'Legionella Management' folder. She has a background knowledge of what is required from her induction training but wants to ensure the checks are carried out correctly. Which one of the options listed is a document held on the premises that should provide the information required to complete this task?

7. At the end of a busy day, a member of staff has got changed and rushed down the stairs ready to leave for home but slipped and fallen while doing so. Unfortunately, she has injured her wrist and is taken to hospital for treatment by a colleague. Which one of the options listed is the set of regulations that will determine whether her employer is required to report the incident to the Health and Safety Executive (HSE) or not?

8. As a new member of the dental team following qualification as a dental nurse, a colleague has been told that she will have several practical duties as an operator involved with the exposure and processing of radiographs. She is asked to position a film in a patient's mouth, ready for exposure, but believes that this task is beyond her current qualification level and so refuses to do so. Which two of the options listed are documents that should be consulted by the colleague and her employer to clarify the matter?

Answers

Multiple choice questions

1. *The correct answer is C.* Health Technical Memorandum 04-01 gives guidance on the actions required to ensure that patients are not exposed to contaminated water supplies while undergoing dental treatment on the premises. It follows the Health and Safety Executive's approved code of conduct (ACOP L8) for the prevention of Legionella contamination in the dental unit waterlines.
2. *The correct answer is D.* Under these regulations it is a legal requirement for dental employers to provide certain items of PPE for their staff, to prevent them coming into contact with blood and other bodily fluids during their normal working day. Following the coronavirus pandemic of 2020–2021, dental staff undertaking aerosol-generating procedures are also currently required to wear enhanced PPE, especially a fit-tested high-grade respirator mask or hood.
3. *The correct answer is C.* This publication enshrines the core principles of being a dental professional and is intended for use by all members of the dental team, both before and after qualification and by whichever category of training, qualification and registration is being followed.
4. *The correct answer is B.* In line with the Ionising Radiation Regulations 2017, the legal person must be the employer or business owner and they have a legal responsibility for implementing the requirements of the regulations.
5. *The correct answer is D.* Knowledge of a subject is gained by learning about it, such as in lectures and other learning-based events, or by experience, such as that gained by working in the dental workplace. In this environment the student can observe qualified colleagues carrying out their day-to-day duties before being trained 'hands-on' to carry out those duties, while completing their Record of Experience document.
6. *The correct answer is D.* Since this Order came into being it has been a legal requirement for all dental registrants to have indemnity insurance in place throughout their career. So not just dentists but all groups of dental care professionals must make an annual declaration to the General Dental Council that they have indemnity in place, otherwise they cannot remain on the register.
7. *The correct answer is A.* This Order gradually brought all dental care professionals under the regulatory umbrella of the General Dental Council, so that all groups wishing to work in the dental professions have to undertake compulsory training and qualification to do so. A period of grandparenting allowed unqualified but well-experienced dental nurses to join the register without prior qualification until 2008.
8. *The correct answer is D.* Dentistry and dental nursing are professions that undergo continual change, development and improvement. The knowledge

and skills required to deliver successful dental and nursing care are continually changing and progressing, so those learnt by initial qualification are, to some extent, now obsolete. New skills and knowledge of new techniques and materials can only be acquired if dental staff undertake lifelong learning in their particular profession. This is the purpose of continuing professional development activities and the reason why they are compulsory.

9. *The correct answer is B.* These regulations require employers to carry out a risk assessment to identify systems that need to be in place to avoid muscle and eye strain, fatigue and headaches in all staff using display screens on their premises.

10. *The correct answer is D.* A Legionella outbreak is considered a serious incident that could result in serious injury or death. It is classed as a significant event and must therefore be reported to the Health and Safety Executive as a notifiable incident, under the Reporting of Injuries, Diseases and Dangerous Occurrences Regulations (RIDDOR) 2013. The Water Supply (Water Fittings) Regulations 1999 are concerned with ensuring that the mains water supply is not contaminated by back-siphonage from the dental premises.

11. *The correct answer is A.* Health Technical Memorandum 01-05 is the relevant guidance in England, with national variations available for Wales, Northern Ireland and Scotland. All dental workplaces should hold a full copy of the document and all staff should have access to it and undergo regular update training in its contents.

12. *The correct answer is D.* Health Technical Memorandum 07-01 is the specific guidance about the safe management of healthcare waste in the dental sector, issued by the Department of Health and the Environment Agency. It contains information on waste segregation using a colour-coding system that applies to all healthcare waste producers, not just dental producers. This allows easy recognition of stored waste by those handling it.

13. *The correct answer is E.* The Reporting of Injuries, Diseases and Dangerous Occurrences Regulations (RIDDOR) require employers to notify the Health and Safety Executive of major accidents and dangerous occurrences that have happened on the premises and accidents that cause more than 7 days absence from work for an employee. Amongst the dangerous occurrences that must be reported is the explosion of a pressure vessel, either an autoclave or an air compressor in the dental workplace.

Extended matching questions

1. *The correct answer is d).* This document itemises the safe and correct segregation of healthcare waste and will inform the workplace that new purple-topped yellow waste receptacles are required for the safe disposal of cytotoxic waste products, such as Botox syringes.

2. *The correct answer is f).* The Ionising Radiation Regulations 2017 are concerned with the safety of staff while on the premises where X-rays are in use and with ensuring the correct functioning of the X-ray equipment. IR(ME)R 2017 are concerned with the safety of patients while on the premises and during their exposure to X-rays.

3. *The correct answer is b).* This document provides full guidance on all aspects of decontamination in primary care dental workplaces, including the recommended tests to be carried out on various items of decontamination equipment.

4. *The correct answer is j).* All members of the dental team should have access to the General Dental Council's *Standards for the Dental Team* document, either as a hard copy or accessible online at the GDC's website. It enshrines the regulator's expectations of the dental team as professionals in society and lays out the 'dos' and 'don'ts' of working as a successful dental professional. Principle 8 (raise concerns if patients are at risk) clearly states in standard 8.1.2 that dental professionals 'must not enter into a contract or agreement which contains a gagging clause. . .' as this would prevent them from always putting patients' safety first.

5. *The correct answer is a).* All dental workplaces should have a COSHH folder on the premises with details of every chemical and hazardous substance used, including the first aid actions to take in the event of an injury to a staff member or a patient by one of the substances.

6. *The correct answer is c).* This document will give information on the temperature ranges required for both the hot and cold water supplies, to ensure that if achieved, Legionella should be prevented from contaminating the workplace.

7. *The correct answer is h).* The injuries that must be reported to HSE under RIDDOR are listed in the document and include fracture of the long bone of an arm. If the injury is less severe, such as a sprained wrist, the injury need not be reported but should be recorded in the accident book at the workplace. An internal investigation should be carried out to determine how the injury occurred and how similar events can be avoided in the future.

8. *The correct answers are e) and i).* The former set of regulations lay out the roles and responsibilities of the various dental personnel involved in taking and processing radiographs within the workplace and will confirm that only dental nurses with an appropriate post-registration qualification in radiography are able to position the film. The General Dental Council's *Scope of Practice* document will list this task as one able to be carried out by dental nurses holding a suitable post-registration qualification in dental radiography and not by other dental nurses.

INDEX

Questions and Answers for Dental Nurses, Fourth Edition. Carole Hollins.